LASERS AND ELECTRO-OPTICS RESEARCH AND TECHNOLOGY

MICROBIOCHIPS MONOLITHICALLY INTEGRATED WITH MICROFLUIDICS, MICROMECHANICS, PHOTONICS, AND ELECTRONICS BY 3D FEMTOSECOND LASER DIRECT WRITING

LASERS AND ELECTRO-OPTICS RESEARCH AND TECHNOLOGY

Additional books in this series can be found on Nova's website at:
https://www.novapublishers.com/catalog/index.php?cPath=23_29&
seriesp=Lasers+and+ElectroOptics+Research+and+
Technology

Additional E-books in this series can be found on Nova's website at:
https://www.novapublishers.com/catalog/index.php?cPath=23_29&
seriespe=Lasers+and+ElectroOptics+Research+and+
Technology

LASERS AND ELECTRO-OPTICS RESEARCH AND TECHNOLOGY

MICROBIOCHIPS MONOLITHICALLY INTEGRATED WITH MICROFLUIDICS, MICROMECHANICS, PHOTONICS, AND ELECTRONICS BY 3D FEMTOSECOND LASER DIRECT WRITING

YA CHENG
KOJI SUGIOKA
KATSUMI MIDORIKAWA
AND
ZHIZHAN XU

Novinka
Nova Science Publishers, Inc.
New York

Copyright © 2010 by Nova Science Publishers, Inc.

All rights reserved. No part of this book may be reproduced, stored in a retrieval system or transmitted in any form or by any means: electronic, electrostatic, magnetic, tape, mechanical photocopying, recording or otherwise without the written permission of the Publisher.

For permission to use material from this book please contact us:
Telephone 631-231-7269; Fax 631-231-8175
Web Site: http://www.novapublishers.com

NOTICE TO THE READER

The Publisher has taken reasonable care in the preparation of this book, but makes no expressed or implied warranty of any kind and assumes no responsibility for any errors or omissions. No liability is assumed for incidental or consequential damages in connection with or arising out of information contained in this book. The Publisher shall not be liable for any special, consequential, or exemplary damages resulting, in whole or in part, from the readers' use of, or reliance upon, this material.

Independent verification should be sought for any data, advice or recommendations contained in this book. In addition, no responsibility is assumed by the publisher for any injury and/or damage to persons or property arising from any methods, products, instructions, ideas or otherwise contained in this publication.

This publication is designed to provide accurate and authoritative information with regard to the subject matter covered herein. It is sold with the clear understanding that the Publisher is not engaged in rendering legal or any other professional services. If legal or any other expert assistance is required, the services of a competent person should be sought. FROM A DECLARATION OF PARTICIPANTS JOINTLY ADOPTED BY A COMMITTEE OF THE AMERICAN BAR ASSOCIATION AND A COMMITTEE OF PUBLISHERS.

LIBRARY OF CONGRESS CATALOGING-IN-PUBLICATION DATA

Available upon Request
ISBN: 978-1-61728-279-9

Published by Nova Science Publishers, Inc. ✝ *New York*

Contents

Preface		**vii**
Chapter 1	Introduction	1
Chapter 2	Concept of 3D Direct Writing Inside Transparent Materials by Femtosecond Laser	5
Chapter 3	Femtosecond Laser Fabrication of 3D Functional Components	9
Chapter 4	Monolithic Integration of Microfluidics, Photonics, and Electronics	33
Chapter 5	Nanoaquarium for Dynamic Observation of Microorganisms	47
Chapter 6	Conclusions and Outlook	55
References		59
Index		63

PREFACE

Microbiochips, such as a lab-on-a-chip (LOC) devices and micro total analysis systems, can be regarded conceptually as a biological equivalent of conventional silicon integrated circuits, which involve miniaturization and integration of electronics. As its name implies, an ideal LOC should have a very small footprint and yet still be capable of functioning as a laboratory in which partial or complete chemical or biological analysis can be performed automatically. This new book provides an overview of 3D femtosecond laser direct writing technology and highlight its potential for fabrication of complex smart microsystems by furnishing some examples of fabrication and hybrid integration of microfluidics, micromechanics, photonics, and electronics.

Chapter 1

INTRODUCTION

ABSTRACT

Microbiochips such as a lab-on-a-chip (LOC) devices and micro total analysis systems (μ-TAS) can be regarded conceptually as a biological equivalent of conventional silicon integrated circuits, which involve miniaturization and integration of electronics. As its name implies, an ideal LOC should have a very small footprint and yet still be capable of functioning as a laboratory in which partial or complete chemical or biological analysis can be performed automatically. A planar silicon chip that integrates only microelectronics is clearly far from adequate for such a purpose, and other functional components such as microfluidics, microoptics, and micromechanics need to be incorporated into a chip with 3D configurations. This poses a formidable challenge, because current mainstream microfabrication technologies mostly rely on optical lithography, which is essentially a surface structuring technology. Recently, femtosecond laser direct writing has exhibited great potential for producing a variety of true 3D microstructures in various transparent materials. This is enabled by the nonlinear interaction between the tightly focused femtosecond laser beam and the material that is transparent to the laser beam, since the interaction can be effectively confined to the vicinity of focal point where the laser intensity exceeds the threshold for multiphoton absorption. In this book, we provide an overview of 3D femtosecond laser direct writing technology and highlight its potential for fabrication of complex smart microsystems by furnishing some examples of fabrication and hybrid integration of microfluidics, micromechanics, photonics, and electronics. In addition, application of some of our microfluidic chips to biological research has resulted in new insights into various biological behaviors such the dynamics and functions of microorganisms. Possible solutions for overcoming remaining challenges are discussed in the hope that this technology will provide a manufacturing solution for the emerging LOC industry.

Keywords: femtosecond laser direct writing, 3D microfabrication, lab-on-a-chip, microfluidics, micromechanics, photonics, electronics, integrated microchip.

The field of lab-on-a-chip (LOC) technology has experienced tremendous growth over the last few years. A LOC device is a miniaturized system that integrates one or more laboratory functions for chemical and biological analyses. Because of its compact dimensions and high functionality, a LOC device allows chemical and biological analyses to be performed easily with low sample and reagent consumptions, low waste production, rapid analysis, and high reproducibility due to standardization and automation [1,2]. Although LOC technology has been used for a broad range of applications in a variety of fields including medicine, healthcare, pharmaceutics, environmental monitoring, and national security, it is not yet mature and it is still under active development. One major problem is the lack of appropriate technology for fabricating LOC. For example, enclosed microfluidic structures such as microfluidic channels and chambers are key elements in almost all LOC devices; however, because of their inherently 3D nature, they cannot be formed directly inside transparent substrates by 2D microfabrication techniques. To overcome this problem, open microchannels and/or chambers must be initially formed on the surfaces of substrates by photolithography or soft lithography [3~–5], and then stacking and bonding procedures must be used. This leads to additional cost and complexity. On the other hand, unlike semiconductor chips, which mostly consist of just integrated microelectronics, LOC chips are hybrid integrated systems that incorporate elements having different functions. Currently, a common way of achieving monolithic integration of multifunctional components is to first separately fabricate the different types of components and then assemble them onto a substrate using microassembly techniques. However, because of the rapid development of LOC technology, LOC systems are now becoming increasingly complex, making assembly and packaging very difficult, if not impossible. Thus, new fabrication processes need to be developed to tackle these problems.

In this book, we demonstrate that 3D femtosecond laser direct writing has great potential for fabricating LOC devices [6,7]. On the one hand, it allows for direct formation of hollow 3D microstructures embedded in transparent materials without employing any stacking or bonding procedures; such microstructures can serve as microfluidic, microoptical, and micromechanical elements, etc. On the other hand, with this technique, monolithic integration of multifunctional components into a single chip can be realized after a single continuous laser writing process followed by chemical treatments. Since the chemical treatments are batch processes, the increase in the cost of individual LOC chips is insignificant and will not pose a major problem [8].

This book is organized as follows: we begin by providing a brief introduction to the basic concepts of 3D femtosecond laser direct writing in Chapter 2. In Chapter 3, we show how to fabricate multifunctional structures embedded in transparent materials with true 3D configurations. In Chapter 4, we present a few examples of monolithically integrated, fully functional microdevices. In Chapter 5, we demonstrate the use of microfluidic chips fabricated by femtosecond laser micromachining for biological applications such as dynamic observation of microorganisms. Finally, we summarize the current major challenges of this technique and discuss possible solutions to some of these problems in Chapter 6.

Chapter 2

CONCEPT OF 3D DIRECT WRITING INSIDE TRANSPARENT MATERIALS BY FEMTOSECOND LASER

Due to its ultrashort pulse duration, peak intensities of over 10^{14} W/cm^2 can easily be attained by a tightly focused femtosecond laser beam even if the pulse energy is only of the order of microjoules or millijoules. At such high intensities, the electric field of the electromagnetic wave can significantly distort the Coulomb potential of most neutral atoms, making the interaction between the light and matter extremely nonlinear [9,10]. For this reason, femtosecond laser microfabrication has several distinct advantages over conventional laser microfabrication techniques that usually employ nanosecond or continuous-wave lasers. The first advantage is that the interaction between a femtosecond laser beam and a transparent material can occur only in the vicinity of the focal point where the peak intensity is sufficiently high to initiate the multiphoton process. This important property lays the foundation for 3D direct writing inside transparent materials with femtosecond laser pulses, because there is virtually no out-of-focus absorption when a femtosecond laser beam is focused into a bulk material. The second advantage is related to the fact that conventional laser microfabrication relies on linear absorption of light. Because materials have complex electronic band structures, lasers that operate at different wavelengths are required for different materials. This is completely unnecessary for femtosecond laser microfabrication because by gradually increasing the peak intensity, the electric field of a femtosecond laser can always be increased to a level that is not negligible compared with the binding field experienced by electrons in transparent materials. The materials are then forced to absorb photons via nonlinear absorption processes. Thus, a variety of materials can be processed using a single femtosecond laser system by tuning the peak intensity. The third advantage is also a result of the ultrashort pulse duration, namely thermal effects in femtosecond laser fabrication are significantly suppressed, particularly when the peak intensity of the laser is controlled to be near the threshold of multiphoton absorption and the repetition rate is sufficiently low (e.g., a few kilohertz or a few tens of kilohertz). Effective suppression of the heat-affected zone permits fine structures with micrometer- or nanometer-scale features to be fabricated by femtosecond lasers. The fourth advantage is that the physical and chemical properties of materials can be finely tuned or even completely altered in a spatially selective manner using femtosecond laser pulses. Mainly as a result of this unique characteristic, 3D femtosecond laser direct writing can integrate multiple functions on a single substrate.

Figure 1 shows a typical layout of the 3D femtosecond laser direct writing systems used in our experiments [11]. In most of our experiments, the laser wavelength is ~800 nm, the pulse width is ~150 fs, and the repetition rate is 1 kHz, although sometimes we used a laser with a wavelength of 800 nm, a pulse width of ~50 fs, and a repetition rate of 1 kHz. To ensure a high beam quality, the original size of the output laser beam is usually reduced to 3 mm using a circular aperture placed before the focusing system. Microscope objectives with numerical apertures (NA) in the range 0.2~0.8 are selected for experiments requiring different fabrication resolutions and working distances, and we typically use a long-working-distance, ×20 objective lens with an NA of 0.46, which can offer a spatial resolution of ~1 μm and a working distance of 1.8 mm. With this working distance, 3D microstructures can be fabricated in a transparent sample at depths greater than 2 mm due to the refractive index of the material being greater than unity. 3D microstructures are generally formed by the direct writing technique by keeping the laser focal spot fixed while translating the sample in 3D space using a precision XYZ stage. The fabrication process is monitored using a charge coupled device (CCD) camera, the output of which is displayed on a PC monitor.

In principle, 3D femtosecond laser direct writing can be performed inside any material that is transparent to the incident beam [6]. However, to realize multiple functions in a single substrate, most of our experiments were performed with a photosensitive glass manufactured by Schott Corporation and sold under the trade name Foturan [8,12]. The history of photosensitive glass and its fabrication commenced half a century ago. Stooky at Corning conducted the earliest work in developing this material in the 1950s [13].

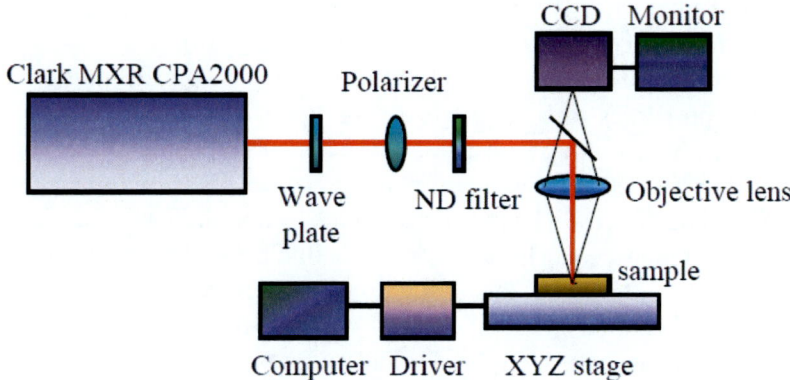

Figure 1. Schematic of a typical system for 3D femtosecond laser direct writing.

The photosensitive glass Foturan is lithium aluminosilicate doped with trace amounts of silver and cerium. The cerium (Ce^{3+}) ion functions as a photosensitizer by absorbing a UV photon at a wavelength near 315 nm and releasing an electron to become Ce^{4+}. Some silver ions then capture some of the free electrons and become silver atoms. In a subsequent heat treatment, the silver atoms diffuse and agglomerate to form nanoclusters at about 500 °C, and then at about 600 °C the crystalline phase of lithium metasilicate grows around the silver clusters (which act as nuclei) in the amorphous glass matrix. This crystalline phase of lithium metasilicate can be preferentially etched since it has a much higher etching rate in dilute hydrofluoric acid than the glass matrix. The conventional exposure procedure for 2D microfabrication on the surface of Foturan glass is a UV lamp photography step. However, to fabricate 3D hollow microstructures in Foturan, it is necessary to focus the laser beam into the sample. Since UV exposure is essentially a single-photon process, the UV beam undergoes linear absorption as it propagates from the glass surface, making internal modification very difficult. In addition, single-photon processes intrinsically have poor fabrication resolutions in the laser beam propagation direction. In contrast, an exposure procedure employing a femtosecond laser can confine the absorption region to an area near the focal spot by using a multiphoton process, improving the axial resolution, which is vital for achieving true 3D microprocessing [14,15]. Our early investigations revealed the photoreaction initiated by multiphoton excitation has a different mechanism from that of single-photon excitation, because the interaction of the high-intensity femtosecond laser with the glass matrix of Foturan generates a large amount of free electrons. Consequently, it is not necessary to dope Foturan glass with cerium for multiphoton processing [16].

In addition, using Foturan glass permits both the chemical etching rate and the optical properties to be controlled. The hollow structures formed inside Foturan usually have rough surfaces, but they can be greatly smoothened for optical components (e.g., micromirrors and microoptical lenses) by a applying a postannealing process [17,18]. Furthermore, since the silver nanoparticles produced by femtosecond laser irradiation exhibit the plasmonic effect, they can be used to tune both the absorption and refractive index of Foturan [19,20]. Thus, Foturan glass is an ideal material for fabricating optofluidic devices, which integrate microfluidics and microoptics in a common substrate [21,22].

Chapter 3

FEMTOSECOND LASER FABRICATION OF 3D FUNCTIONAL COMPONENTS

3.1. MICROFLUIDIC COMPONENTS AND CONTROLLING THE ASPECT RATIO OF MICROCHANNELS

Initially, our research was mainly focused on establishing a technique for directly forming a variety of microfluidic components within glass [14,23,24]. The fabrication process consists of three main steps: (1) 3D direct writing of latent images in the sample using a tightly focused femtosecond laser beam focused using an objective lens, (2) baking the sample in a programmable furnace for the formation of modified regions, and (3) etching the sample in a 10% aqueous solution of hydrofluoric (HF) acid in an ultrasonic bath to selectively remove the modified regions. Figure 2(a) shows X-shaped microfluidic channels formed at a depth of 300 μm below the sample surface with a channel length of ~2800 μm and a width of ~45 μm. The channels appear to be uniform, which is probably a result of using a relatively high concentration of HF acid (10% in our case compared with 5% HF for UV exposure by H. Helvajian et al. [8]) and a high-intensity ultrasonic bath. We find that using an ultrasonic bath is critical for fabricating uniform structures by chemical etching because it greatly enhances the supply of fresh HF acid and reactant in the narrow channels and tiny chambers during etching. Moreover, a chemical microreactor was fabricated by forming microchannels and microchambers with true 3D configurations inside Foturan glass, as shown in Figure 3 [23]. It is noteworthy that all these structures are directly formed in a glass coupon without using any multistep procedures such as stacking and bonding, greatly reducing the cost by enabling high-throughput manufacturing.

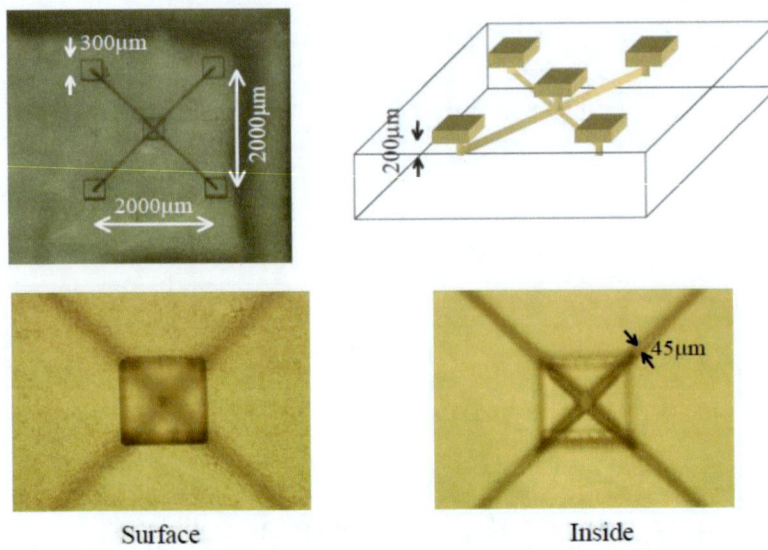

Figure 2. A large-scale crossed-channel buried in Foturan glass.

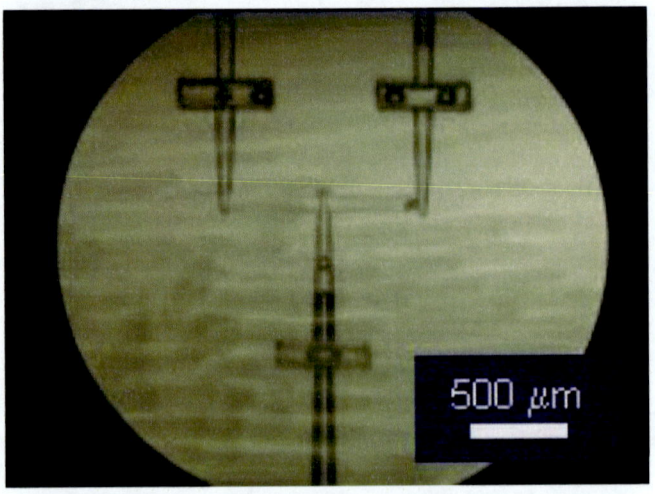

Figure 3. A chemical microreactor with a vertical configuration.

A frequent problem in 3D laser microprocessing is that the vertical resolution (i.e., parallel to the laser beam) is always inferior to the lateral resolution due to the focal spot being elongated in the propagation direction of the laser beam (i.e., the axial direction). Consequently, the cross-sections of fabricated microfluidic channels have high aspect ratios (i.e., the height to width ratio). The cross-section of the Y-branched microfluidic channel in Figure 4 has an aspect ratio of ~4.2 [14]. To overcome this problem, we inserted a narrow slit above the objective lens to tailor the focal spot shape, as illustrated in Figure 5(a). The slit functions as a diffraction aperture and allows the shape of the focal spot and hence the aspect ratio of fabricated channels to be controlled [17]. This is because that the slits causes the laser beam to be loosely focused in the direction perpendicular to the slit, which laterally expands the focal spot; the laser beam will still be tightly focused in the direction parallel to the slit to ensure a high axial resolution. Figure 5(c) shows the cross-section of a microfluidic channel fabricated with a combination of an objective lens with an NA of 0.46 and a 500 μm (width) × 3000 μm (length) slit; it shows that the slit reduces the aspect ratio of the cross-section from ~3 to ~1.6. This technique is also widely used for writing optical waveguides in glasses [25~27]. Using an objective lens with an NA of 0.8 and a slit with dimensions 200 μm (width) × 3000 μm (length) produced waveguides with a completely circular cross-sections (diameter: ~9 μm) that can be used as single-mode waveguides [28].

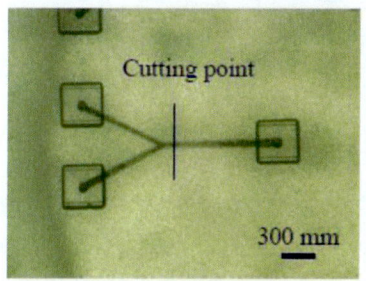

3-D Y-branched structure
fabricated in the photosensitive
glass (focusing on surface)

(a)

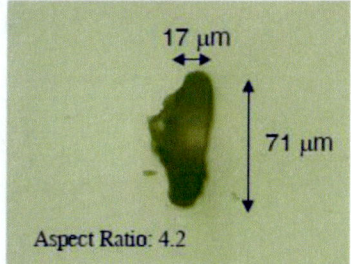

Cross Sectional Shape of
embedded Microchannel

(b)

Figure 4. (a) A horizontal Y-branched microchannel structure embedded 300 μm below the sample surface. (b) Cross-section of the microchannel. The cutting point is indicated in Figure 4(a).

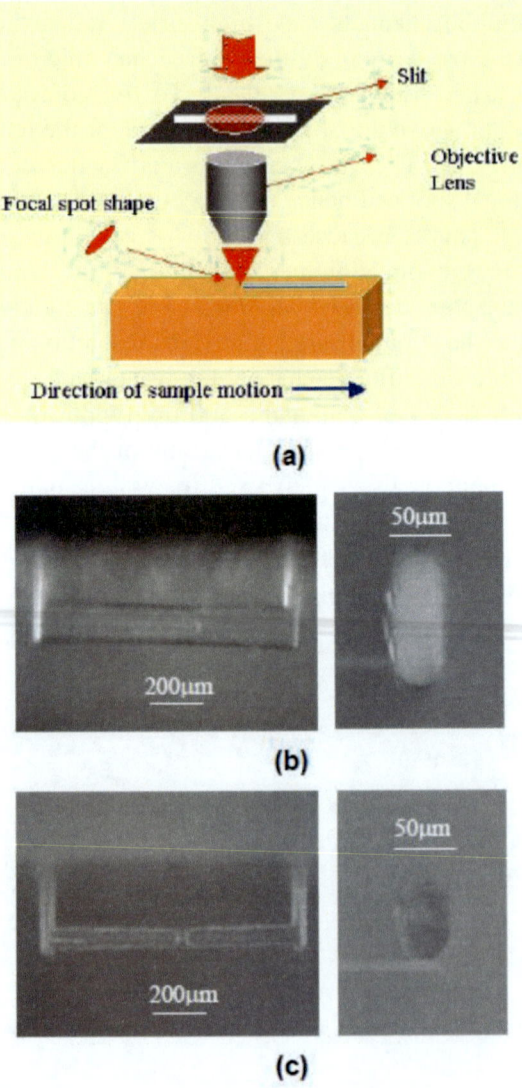

Figure 5. (a) Close-up view of a focusing system with a slit for controlling the microfluidic channel aspect ratio. (b) Side view and cross-section of a bridge-like microstructure fabricated without a slit. (c) Side view and cross-section of the same structure fabricated with a 0.5-mm-wide slit.

Although using a slit to shape the beam can achieve symmetrical cross-sections when fabricating microfluidic channels, it is not the only solution to the problem. In fact, after being shaped by the narrow slit, the focal spot will not be truly spherical in 3D space, but instead it be compressed in the direction parallel to the slit. Compression of the focal spot in the direction parallel to the slit should not be a problem when fabricating 1D microstructures, such as microfluidic channels or optical waveguides, because it can be compensated by reducing the laser scanning speed in the sample; however, an anisotropic focal spot is undesirable in many applications (e.g., 3D data storage in glass using femtosecond laser generated microvoids). In such cases, a three-dimensionally isotropic focal spot is preferable. This can be achieved by using a novel focusing geometry in which two focused femtosecond laser beams are perpendicular to each other [29]. Figure 6(a) shows a schematic view of the crossed-beam irradiation system; the combined optical fields of the two beams results in an isotropic energy distribution in the central region of the focal spot (the area enclosed by the dashed red circle in Figure 6(b)). To ensure an isotropic illumination volume, the foci of the two beams in the crossed-beam system must spatiotemporally overlap throughout the entire period of laser scanning. This is impossible to fulfill if we scan the glass in air due to the mismatch in the refractive indices of Foturan glass ($n\sim1.52$) and air ($n\sim1$). To overcome this problem, we designed a special XYZ stage which translates the glass sample in a refractive index matching liquid, as shown in Figure 6(a).

The liquid is a mixture of α-bromnaphtalene ($n\sim1.66$) and paraffin ($n\sim1.48$); thus, an identical refractive index to that of Foturan glass can be achieved by mixing the two liquids in the appropriate ratio. Since translating the glass sample in a fixed glass cell containing the refractive index matching liquid will not alter the optical paths of the two orthogonal beams, two foci that are initially aligned will continue to spatiotemporally overlap each other over the entire scanning step. Before we started to scan the sample, the two objective lenses were aligned by observing femtosecond-laser-induced fluorescence in the glass sample. That is, when two high-intensity femtosecond laser beams were simultaneously sent into the two objective lenses with a crossed-beam focusing system, two lines of fluorescence were simultaneously observed on the PC monitor connected to a CCD camera. The CCD camera was installed with its optical axis perpendicular to the plane defined by the two crossed beams. We carefully adjusted the positions of the objective lenses using a computer-controlled translation stage to make the centers of the two fluorescence lines spatially overlap.

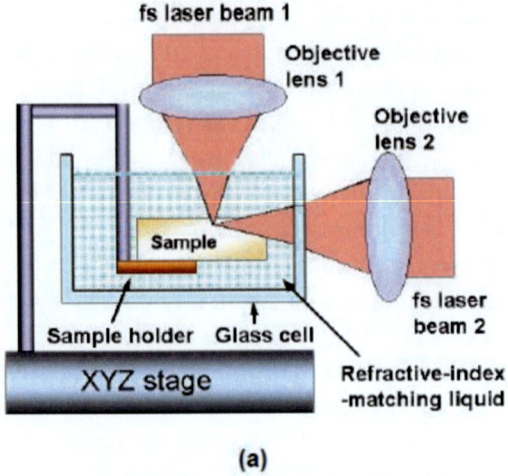

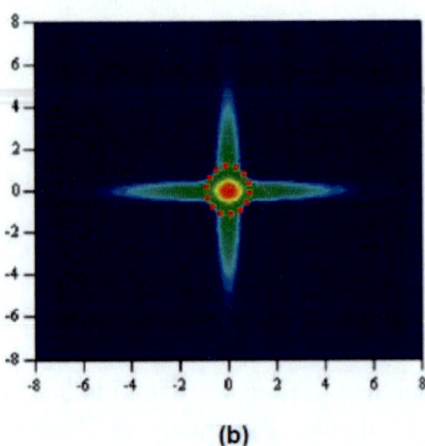

Figure 6. (a) Schematic view of crossed-beam irradiation system. (b) The energy distribution in the focal spot synthesized by the two perpendicular beams.

We then adjusted the time delay between the two beams by varying the optical path length using another translation stage until the fluorescence in the overlapping region of the two fluorescence lines was maximized. When this alignment procedure was completed the crossed-beam irradiation system was able to create microstructures inside glass with isotropic 3D resolution.

To demonstrate the effectiveness of the crossed-beam irradiation geometry, we fabricated several microfluidic channels by both single-beam and crossed-beam irradiation methods, and scanned the samples in different directions. Figures 7(a) and b) clearly show that with single-beam irradiation, the fabricated channel has an elliptical cross-section.

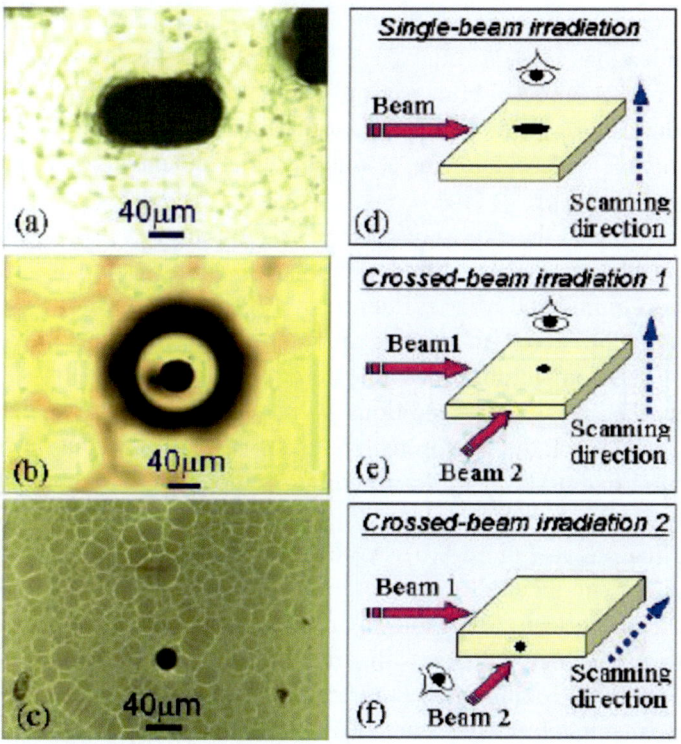

Figure 7. Optical micrographs of the cross-sectional shapes of the microfluidic hollow channels fabricated by (a) single-beam irradiation, (b) crossed-beam irradiation with the laser scanning direction perpendicular to the plane defined by the two beams, and (c) crossed-beam irradiation with the laser scanning direction along the axis of one of the two crossed beams. The scanning geometries for fabricating the structures in (a)c) are presented in (d)f), respectively.

In contrast, when the crossed-beam irradiation method was adopted, the cross-sections of the fabricated microchannels were circular regardless of the scanning direction (see Figures 7(c)f)). The circular cross-section generated at arbitrary scanning directions is clear evidence that a nearly spherical focal spot was generated inside the Foturan glass sample. We believe that this will be very useful in a broad range of applications, including 3D data storage and photonic crystal fabrication by two-photon polymerization [30].

3.2. MICROMECHANICS

Micromechanical structures such as micropumps and active microvalves are important elements for realizing microfluidic routing and switching in LOC applications [14,31,32]. The 3D femtosecond laser direct writing technique allows direct fabrication of mechanical elements encapsulated in a microfluidic cavity. As an example, we first demonstrated the fabrication of a freely movable microplate in a microfluidic chamber that serves as a microvalve (see Figure 8) [14].

Figure 8 shows the exposure scheme in Foturan glass used to fabricate the freely movable microplate. After scanning the femtosecond laser beam at a velocity of 2 mm/s and a laser fluence of 170 mJ/cm^2 in the dark regions in Figure 8(a), the above-mentioned postannealing was performed to form modified regions of lithium metasilicate crystallites. To obtain a high spatial resolution, the irradiation conditions were set slightly above the threshold fluence above which the photosensitive glass was modified but below which it was not modified at all [14]. The modified regions were completely removed in the subsequent chemical wet etching so that hollow structures (indicated by the white regions in Figure 8(b)) were formed in the glass. A movable glass plate was left in the hollow structure, which can serve as a microfluidic chamber. The fabricated movable microplate can function as a microvalve in the microfluidic network, as illustrated in Figure 9. This device was manufactured by stacking three Foturan glass substrates, each with a thickness of 2 mm (the thickest substrate available). A syringe was used as an air compressor to drive the microplate motion. The top layer contains three inlet cells; the center cell is an opening for adding the reagents while the left and right cells are openings attached to silicon tubes for infusing compressed air from the syringes. In the middle layer, a movable microplate was embedded in a rectangular hollow chamber connected to five microchannels to the cells in the top and bottom plates. The microplate was fabricated by the exposure scheme shown in Figure 8. In the bottom layer, two cells were installed in the glass as outlets for the reagents. Each structure was fabricated by the same procedure using the femtosecond laser. The microplate was driven to the right when compressed air was infused from the left opening in the top layer. In this case, the flow channel of the reagents to the right outlet was switched off so that the reagents could flow only to the left outlet (Figure 9(a)). When the compressed air infusion was changed to the right opening, the microplate was driven to the left. As a result, the reagent flow was switched to the right outlet

(Figure 9(b)). Thus, this microplate can switch the flow direction of the reagent like a microvalve.

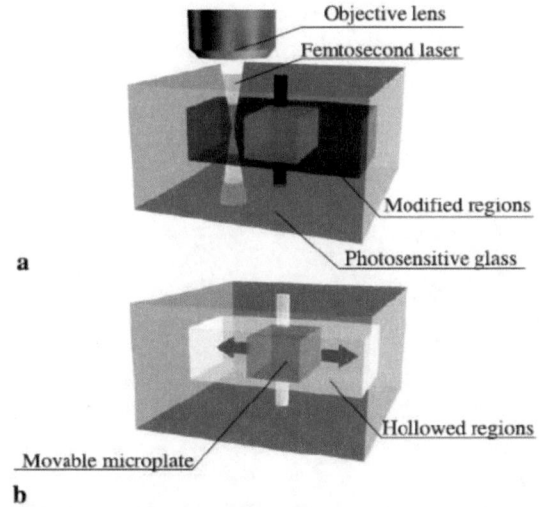

Figure 8. Schematic illustration of the femtosecond laser exposure for fabricating a freely movable microplate embedded in glass. (a) The dark regions are scanned by the focused femtosecond laser beam. (b) The dark regions are completely removed after postannealing and subsequent chemical etching in an HF solution. The movable glass plate is left in the hollow chamber buried in the glass (the white regions).

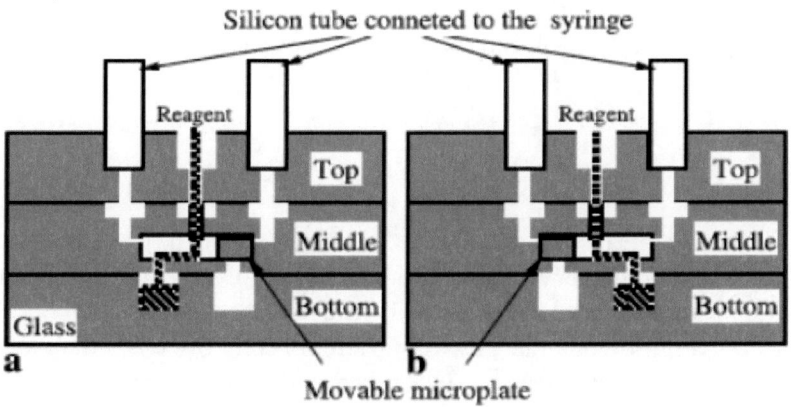

Figure 9. Schematic illustration of the microplate functioning as a microvalve in a microreactor.

Figure 10 shows two photographs of the fabricated sample. It is clear that the microplate moves from one side to another when the infusion direction of the compressed air is switched. We confirmed that the microvalve can switch the flow direction of microfluids by injecting a liquid into the microdevice. More recently, a freely movable micromechanical needle was integrated into a microfluidic biochip to elucidate the information transmission process in Pleurosira laevis [32].

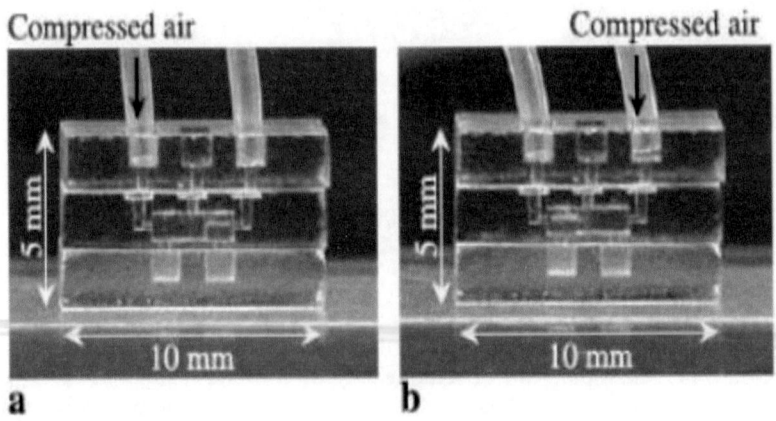

Figure 10. Photographs of a fabricated microreactor in which a freely movable microplate is embedded. (a) When compressed air was infused from the left opening in the top layer, the microplate moved to the right side. (b) When the infusion of the compressed air was changed to the right opening, the microplate moved to the left side.

3.3. MICROOPTICS

Since chemical and biological analyses frequently employ optical detection methods, integration of microoptics into LOC chips has advantages such as low cost, robustness, stability, and ease of operation [33]. The microstructuring of Foturan glass by a femtosecond laser is essentially non-ablative processing that results in smooth and debris-free internal surfaces; thus, both 3D microfluidic components and 3D microoptics can be simultaneously fabricated inside the glass. For example, Figure 11(a) shows a 45° micromirror embedded in Foturan glass [17]. To fabricate this structure, we scanned parallel lines layer by layer from the top surface to the bottom of the sample. The interval between two adjacent lines in the Foturan glass was set at ~15 μm. Thus, since the total sample thickness was 2000 μm, we scanned 140 parallel lines to form a plane structure vertically embedded in glass. The laser pulse energy was 700 nJ and the scanning speed was 500 μm/s. After laser irradiation, the sample was subjected to heat treatment and then to chemical etching. In this case, chemical etching was performed for about ~1 h. Finally, we rinsed the sample in distilled water and dried it with nitrogen gas flow. To examine the optical properties of the micromirror, we polished the four sidewalls of the glass sample. We then examined the beam spot produced by reflecting a helium-neon (He-Ne) laser beam from the etched internal surface. An incident angle of 45° resulted in total reflection. The two arrows in Figure 11(a) indicate the optical path. A receiving screen was placed 10 mm from the end of the Foturan glass. The arrow head in Figure 11(b) indicates the reflected beam spot on this screen. The beam spot was significantly larger than the incident laser beam, indicating that the reflected beam is highly divergent. Since the lithium metasilicate crystallites developed by postannealing must grow to a certain size (a few microns) to form an etchable network, etching of the crystallites naturally leaves a rough surface. This high roughness causes strong scattering and consequently the reflected light beam is highly divergent and has a high loss. Therefore, it is essential to reduce the surface roughness for microoptical applications. We overcame this problem by including an additional annealing process. After chemical etching, we baked the Foturan glass sample again. The temperature of this additional annealing was lower than that used to crystallize lithium metasilicate. In this annealing process, the sample was heated to 570 °C at 5 °C/min, it was held at this temperature for 5 h, and then cooled to 370 °C at 1 °C/min. After the sample cooled to room temperature, we reexamined its optical properties. The results are shown in Figure 11(c). The reflected beam spot is clearly much smaller than that from the sample that was not subjected to the additional annealing, which demonstrates that the divergence of reflected beam has been reduced. Figures 12(a) and (b) show the morphologies of etched surfaces that had not and had been subjected to the additional annealing, respectively.

Figure 12(b) reveals that after the additional annealing, the smoothness of surface is comparable to that of a polished glass surface (although there are still a few irregular nanodots on the surface). The average surface roughness before the additional annealing was measured to be ~81 nm, whereas after the annealing it was only ~0.8 nm. Consequently, both the divergence angle and the optical loss of the reflected beam can be reduced.

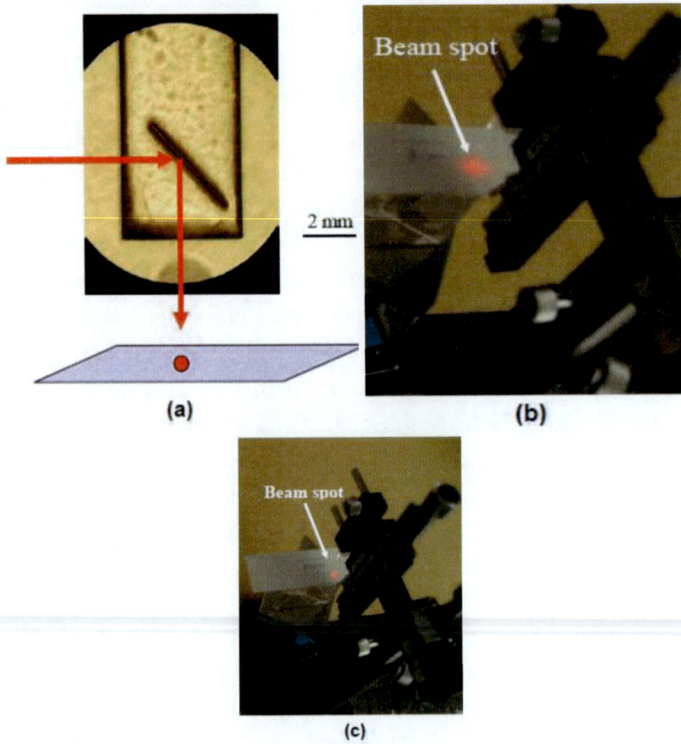

Figure 11. (a) Top view of the 3D micromirror fabricated inside Foturan glass with its optical path indicated by arrows. Beam spots reflected from the sample (b) before and (c) after the additional annealing.

In addition to microoptical structures with plane surfaces, microlenses with curved surfaces can be produced using this technique [18]. Microlenses are important elements for optical biosensors, and they are used as collimators, focusers, and imaging elements [34]. Figures 13(a) and (b) show respectively a microoptical cylindrical lens and a hemispherical lens fabricated on Foturan glass by 3D femtosecond laser direct writing; the focal spots produced by these lenses are shown on the right. These microlenses were fabricated by gouging them out from the Foturan matrix, but they can be also formed inside the glass chip by the present technique for fabricating hollow microstructures [35].

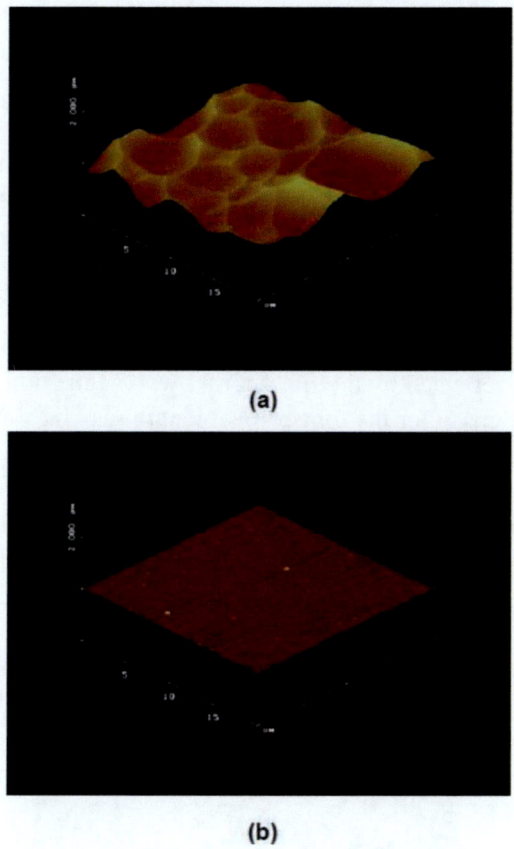

(a)

(b)

Figure 12. AFM images of the surface of Foturan glass after the irradiation by the femtosecond laser beam and chemical etching (a) before and (b) after the additional annealing.

The fabricated hollow structures have openings at one or both ends in a Foturan glass chip and one of the internal sidewalls of the hollow structure is spherical in shape, (i.e., it has a plano-concave hollow structure), as shown in Figure 14. The curvature of the spherical surface corresponds exactly to the designed optical microlens curvature so that the curved surface can function as a plano-convex lens. Thus, a microoptical lens can be fabricated inside a glass chip. Figure 14 also shows optical microscope images of a plano-convex microlens fabricated inside a glass chip with a thickness of 2 mm, a radius of curvature R of 0.75 mm (designed value), and a focal length of 1.5 mm (calculated using the formula: $1/f = (n-1)(1/R)$, $n=1.5$ (refractive index of photosensitive glass)). The figure shows that one of the sidewalls of the buried hollow structure is spherical in shape with a smooth surface, although a small bump is visible on the lens surface. To examine the focusing performance of the microlens, we irradiated a He–Ne laser beam such that it passed through the microlens inside the glass, and the focused laser beam was projected onto a CCD camera by a ×20 objective lens with an NA of 0.35. The focal spot size was approximately 30 µm in diameter for an incident He–Ne laser beam of Φ1.5–1.8 mm. Furthermore, we roughly estimated the focal length experimentally and found that it was about 1.7 mm. This focal length is slightly longer than the designed value of 1.5 mm. Reflection at the air–glass interface is probably responsible for the longer focal length; in other words, the laser beam is reflected by the flat internal wall of the hollow structure after the lens. Another cause for the longer focal length may be somewhat imperfect fabrication precision. The efficiency of the fabricated microlens was evaluated to be more than 80%. The optical loss is considered to be mainly due to four Fresnel reflections at the air–glass interfaces (two glass chip sidewalls and two lens surfaces). Subtracting the loss of the four Fresnel reflections (4% for each), the net loss is estimated to be ~6%. However, the focusing results and the efficiency evaluation indicate that the smooth spherical surface of the buried hollow structure is suitable for optical applications.

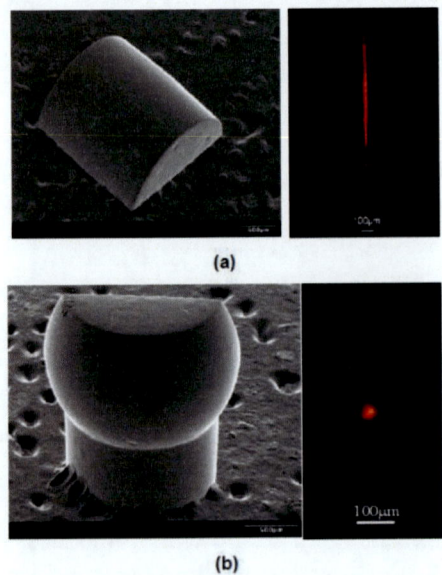

Figure 13. SEM images of microoptical (a) cylindrical and (b) hemispherical lenses. The focal spots produced both lenses are presented in the right panel.

By using 3D femtosecond laser direct writing, microoptical and photonic components have now been fabricated in various transparent materials by modifying their refractive indices [6,20,36]. Changes in the refractive index can be induced in Foturan glass by femtosecond laser irradiation followed by annealing at 520 °C [20]. This results in silver nanoparticles being selectively precipitated in the irradiated region, which changes the refractive index by as much as ~0.4%. Since the process involves only a photochemical reaction, the pulse energy for such processing was as low as 70 nJ/pulse for an objective lens with an NA of 0.8. Such a low pulse energy induced little thermal effects, resulting in a high spatial resolution.

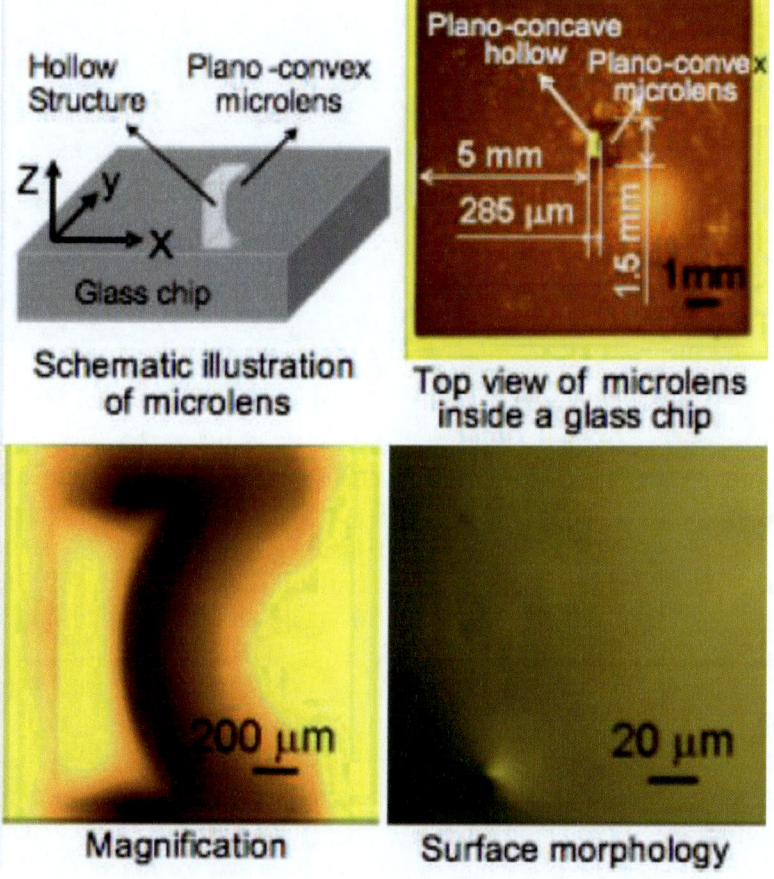

Figure 14. Schematic illustration and optical microscope images of a plano-convex microlens buried in Foturan glass.

Figure 15 shows a 5-μm-pitch micrograting together with its diffraction pattern obtained using a He-Ne laser beam. Using the same principle, optical waveguides can be fabricated inside Foturan glass; guided beams in these waveguides have a single-mode profile because the beam was shaped using a slit during waveguide writing [28].

Very recently, a volume optical grating has been formed inside Foturan glass by focusing a femtosecond laser beam using a pair of cylindrical lenses [37].

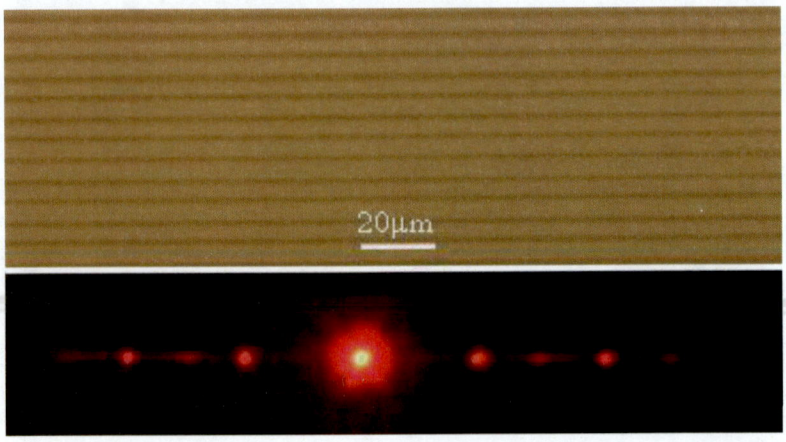

Figure 15. A 5-μm-pitch microoptical grating (upper) embedded in Foturan glass and its diffraction pattern (lower).

In this work, each cylindrical lens focuses the beam in one dimension, so that each femtosecond laser beam pulse forms a vertical plane at the focus. This enables the volume grating to be fabricated by simply translating the sample perpendicular to the cylindrical lens at a constant speed while the laser beam is periodically switched on and off using a programmable shutter. This technique significantly reduces the time required to fabricate a volume grating because there is no need to scan the laser beam parallel to the cylindrical lens.

Even femtosecond laser direct writing without postannealing can increase the refractive index in Foturan glass [38,39]. This process is based on photophysical and/or photothermal reactions such as compaction and direct bond breaking, so it requires much higher pulse **energies** ($\bar{1}2$ μJ/pulse) than femtosecond laser direct writing in Foturan followed by annealing. However, optical waveguides written by this process have higher transmission efficiencies, especially in the visible region, since silver nanoparticles are not precipitated. The propagation loss at 632.8 nm was evaluated by fabricating three waveguides of different lengths under the same conditions in coupons cut out from the same substrate. Figure 16 shows the optical loss as a function of waveguide length for three different scanning speeds. The data were fit with linear equations; the slope of the linear fit represents the propagation loss in decibels per centimeter and the y-axis intercept gives the coupling loss from both facets of the waveguide. The coupling loss is clearly caused by a size mismatch or misalignment between the waveguide and the focused He–Ne laser beam.

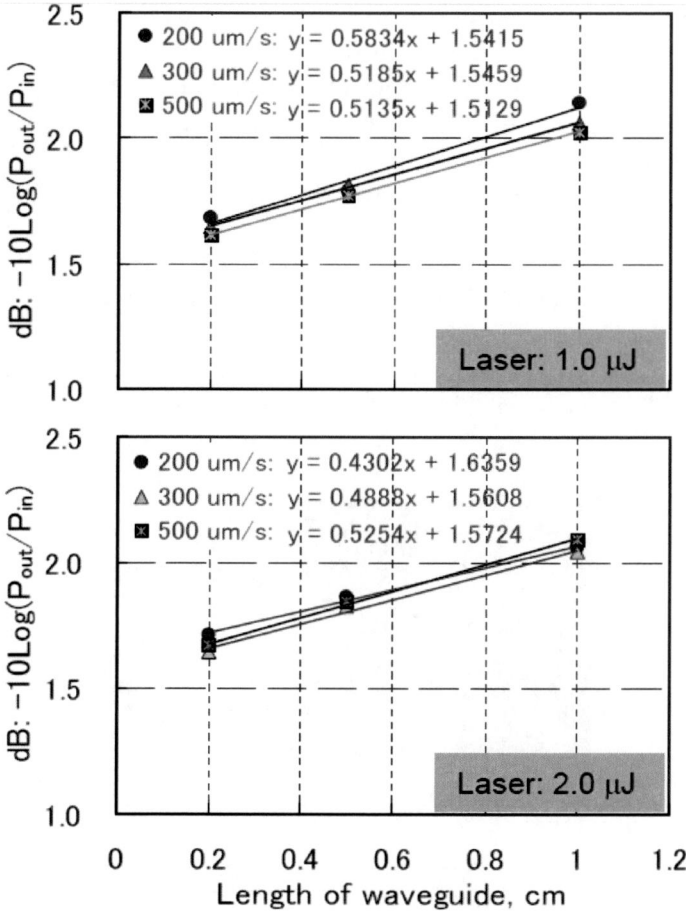

Figure 16. Dependence of optical loss on the length of waveguides written at different laser energies and scanning speeds. Linear fit equations give the propagation loss in dB/cm (slope) and the coupling loss in dB (y-axis intercept).

However, the values obtained under the different conditions in this experiment are quite similar to each other, being in the range 1.5 to 1.6 dB. The propagation loss is around 0.5 dB/cm for all samples under the conditions investigated. This propagation loss is within acceptable limits for biophotonic microchip applications.

Since the physical properties of the photosensitive glass in unirradiated regions did not change markedly even after multiple thermal treatments, we were able to write optical waveguides inside the glass by femtosecond-laser-induced refractive index modification after fabricating 3D hollow structures. Thus, 3D integration of waveguides with microoptics, such as micromirrors and microlenses with hollow structures, can be realized in a single glass chip.

Figure 17 shows an optical microscope image of a microoptical circuit in which two waveguides were integrated by a micromirror and a microlens in a single glass chip. In the fabricated structures, a 5-mm-long waveguide (waveguide I) is connected to a micromirror at an angle of 45° and it is also connected to a 4-mm-long waveguide (waveguide II) at an angle of 90°. The writing of waveguide II was terminated 2 mm before the plano-convex microlens so as to obtain a focused beam output. In order to characterize the 3D integrated microoptical device, we coupled a HeNe laser beam into waveguide I and placed a ×20 objective lens outside the glass chip to capture images of the focused beam spot (indicated by the red arrow in Figure 17) using a CCD camera. In this manner, the near-field focal spot profile was observed.

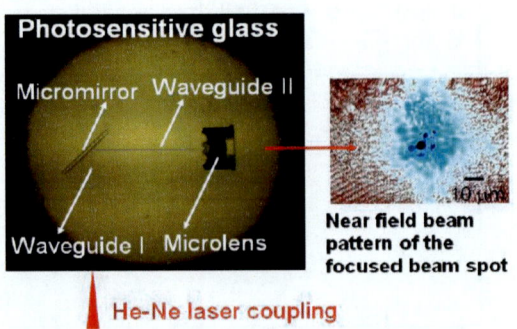

Figure 17. Optical microscope image and characterization of 3D integration of two waveguides with a micromirror and an optical plano-convex microlens in a single glass chip. Solid gray lines indicate the invisible waveguides in the glass.

As seen in Figure 17, the output spot size (dark blue spot) was about 7 μm in diameter. Thus, the combination of a microlens with a waveguide is highly effective for laser beam transmission. As mentioned above, the propagation loss of the optical waveguide was 0.5 dB/cm and the net loss of the microlens was ~6%.

In addition, the bending loss at the micromirror was evaluated to be less than 0.3 dB at a wavelength of 632.8 nm [38]. One of the biggest advantages of this structure is that it can bend a light beam in a small area with a small bending loss. From a practical point of view, a light beam guided by a waveguide often needs to be bent when it is integrated into optical and microfluidic devices. A curved waveguide is commonly used to bend a beam, but its bending loss is significant and cannot be disregarded. To minimize the bending loss, the curvature of a curved waveguide should be greater than several millimeters (e.g., 5–6 mm), but this causes an undesirable increase in the device size. Thus, 3D integration of waveguides with a microlens and a micromirror should enable efficient transmission of a light beam in biophotonic microchip devices.

3.4. MICROELECTRONICS

Fabrication of microelectronic components by femtosecond laser direct writing is certainly desirable for developing monolithic and compact LOC systems [40–45]. Selective metallization of the surfaces of some glass materials (e.g., Foturan and microscope slide glass) has been achieved by direct femtosecond laser ablation followed by electroless copper plating, but this technique cannot be applied to other glass materials such as fused silica [40]. The process requires a certain degree of surface roughness for the so-called "anchor effect" to operate, which enables the deposited metal film to adhesion strongly to the glass surface.

Figure 18 shows optical microscope images of fine metal lines deposited on a Foturan surface after electroless plating. The laser power was varied from 1.2 to 3 mW and the laser scanning speed was 50 μm/s. As an application of this selective metallization technique, Figure 19 shows a microheater that was fabricated on a Foturan glass chip. The microheater temperature is a linear function of the electric power applied to it [40].

With the purpose of realizing selective metallization on surfaces of dielectric materials other than Foturan and microscope slide glass, a modified femtosecond laser direct writing was developed [42–45].

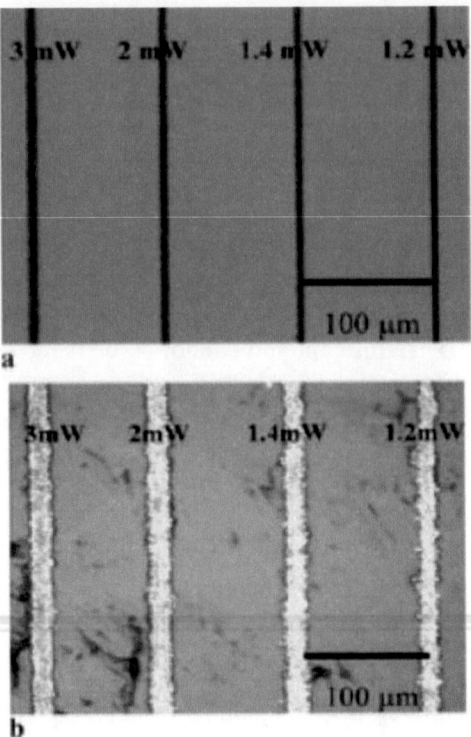

Figure 18. Optical microscope images of (a) as ablated and (b) copper-plated glass after ablation. The laser power is varied from 1.2 to 3 mW. The laser scanning speed is 50 μm/s.

As illustrated in Figure 20, the fabrication process consists of four main steps: (1) formation of silver nitrate thin films on insulator substrates by dip coating, (2) selective modification of insulator surfaces by femtosecond laser direct writing, (3) removal of unirradiated silver nitrate film by acetone, and (4) selective copper coating by electroless plating.

In our experiment, a 3-mm-thick lithium niobate (LiNbO$_3$) crystal was used as the insulator substrate because of its potential application to electro-optic integration [42].

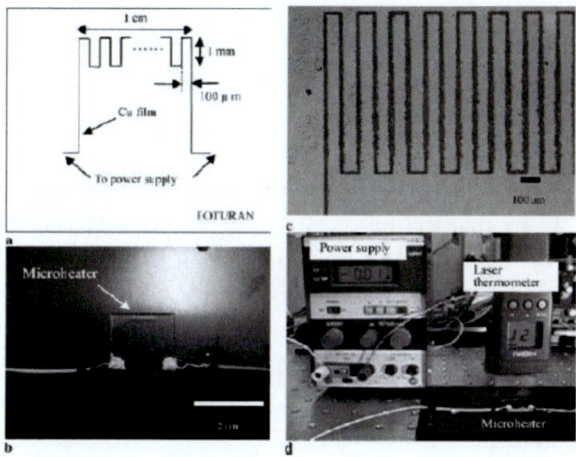

Figure 19. (a) Schematic diagram of a microheater; (b) microscope image of the microheater; (c) enlarged image of the left-hand end of the microheater; (d) experimental setup for measuring the temperature of the microheater.

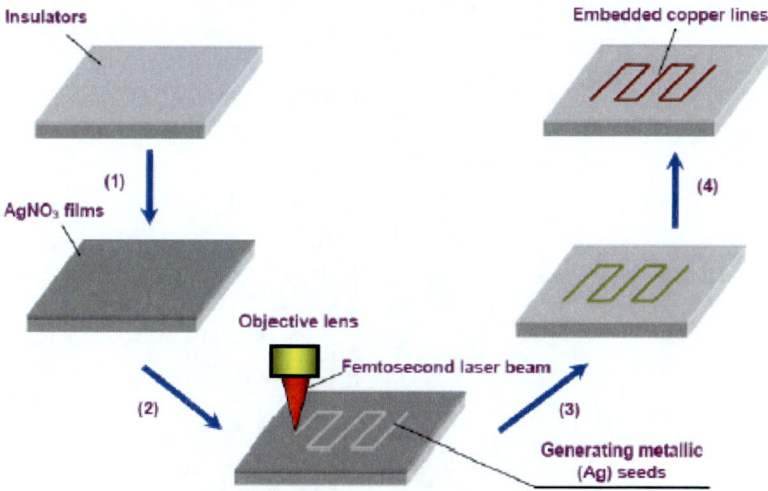

Figure 20. Schematic illustration of the fabrication process for the selective metallization of insulators: (1) formation of silver nitrate thin films on insulator substrates; (2) modification of insulator surfaces by femtosecond laser direct writing; (3) removal of unirradiated silver nitrate films by acetone; (4) copper coating by selective electroless plating.

Figures 21(a) and (b) show top and end view images of electrodes embedded in a crystal, respectively. Two 10-μm-wide grooves with a 16 μm center-to-center interval between them were ablated using a tightly focused femtosecond laser beam with an average power of 10 mW and a scanning speed of 200 μm/s.

The micrograph of the V-shaped cross-section of the electrodes shown in Figure 21(b) reveals that the two ~10-μm-deep grooves have been filled with deposited copper after electroless plating for 120 min. Since optical waveguides can also be directly written inside a LiNbO3 crystal using femtosecond laser pulses [46], the embedded microelectrodes can thus be easily integrated with the buried optical waveguides, opening up the potential to fabricate 3D micro-electro-optical devices such as optical switches and optical modulators.

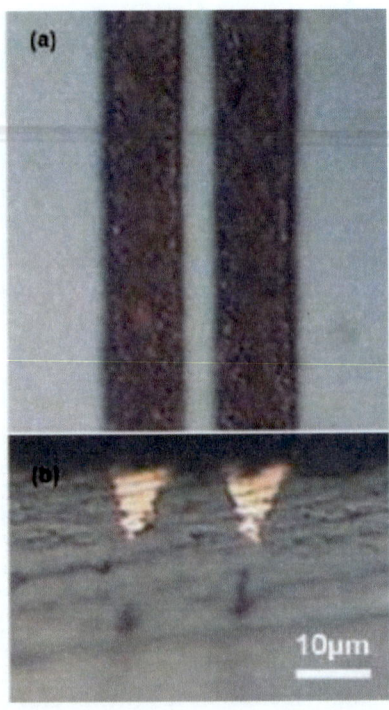

Figure 21. Optical micrographs of microelectrodes embedded in a LiNbO3 crystal: (a) top view and (b) end view.

Although selective metallization of insulators using nanosecond lasers has been reported [47,48], the use of femtosecond lasers has several critical advantages. One advantage is that, as Figure 21(b) clearly shows, the microelectrodes are embedded deep within the insulator, which is a desirable characteristic for many novel microdevices requiring 3D configurations. Another advantage is that when the femtosecond laser intensity is well controlled near the ablation threshold, selective metallization of glass can be realized with a nanometer-scale spatial resolution, as demonstrated by the fact that tiny nanostructures (i.e., nanometer-sized holes and grooves) have been reliably produced in dielectrics using a femtosecond laser [49]. A further advantage of this technique is that it offers the ability to directly incorporate microelectrical elements into microoptical and/or microfluidic circuits in a single glass chip. Future development of this technique holds great promise for rapid, flexible, and cost-effective fabrication of monolithic 3D micro-electro-opto-fluidic devices.

Chapter 4

MONOLITHIC INTEGRATION OF MICROFLUIDICS, PHOTONICS, AND ELECTRONICS

4.1. MICROFLUIDIC DYE LASER

With the establishment of the above-mentioned capabilities, microoptics and microfluidics can be readily integrated into a single glass chip by 3D femtosecond laser direct writing for fabricating hybrid devices. In particular, we are interested in a microfluidic dye laser which is a useful light source for optical analyses such as fluorescence detection or photoabsorption spectroscopy in LOC systems [22].

Figure 22(a) shows a micrograph of the top view of a fabricated microfluidic laser that has an optical microcavity composed of four 45° micromirrors vertically buried in glass, a horizontal microfluidic chamber embedded ~400 μm beneath the glass surface, and a microfluidic through channel that passes through the center of the microchamber.

Figure 22(b) shows a micrograph of the side view of a fabricated microfluidic laser, showing the microchannel that has an average diameter of ~80 μm and the microchamber that is ~200 μm thick. Figure 22(c) depicts the optical path of the microfluidic laser. The optical cavity is composed of a pair of corner mirrors, which are formed by two micromirrors on the left-hand side and two micromirrors on the right-hand side. Light bounces back and forth in the optical cavity by total internal reflection. Lasing can occur if the microchamber is filled with a gain medium laser dye rhodamine 6G (Rh6G) and then pumped by a frequency-doubled Nd:yttrium aluminum garnet (Nd:YAG) laser.

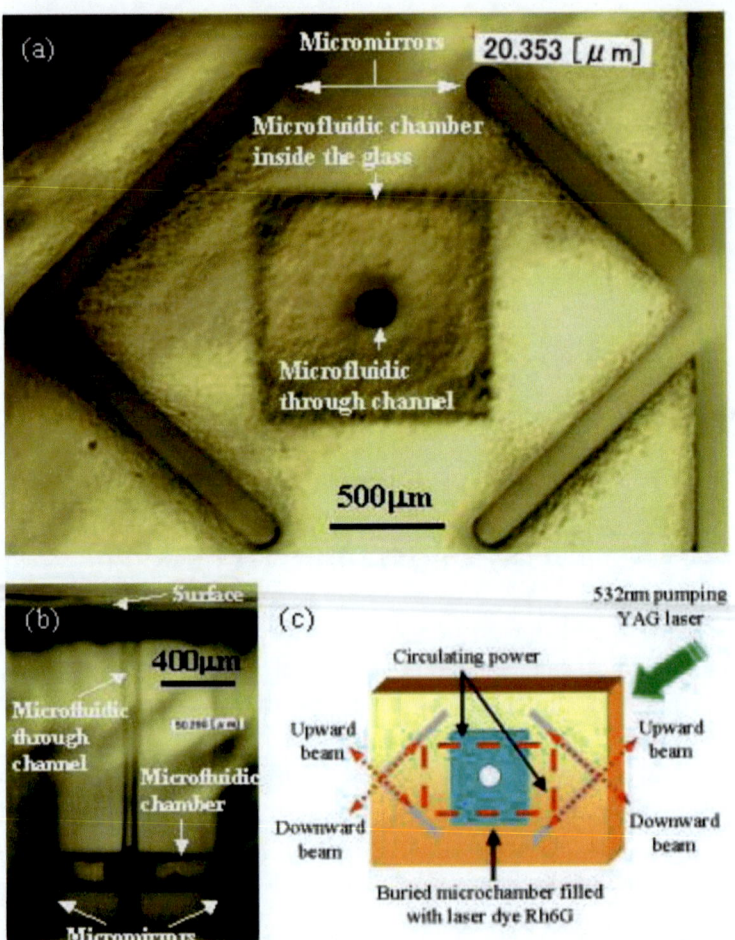

Figure 22. (a) Optical micrographs of the top-view of the microfluidic laser and (b) of the side view of the microfluidic chamber and through channel. (c) The light path in the microfluidic laser.

Since the surfaces of the micromirrors could not be fabricated perfectly smooth, and also the angle between any two micromirrors could not be exactly 90° due to the limited fabrication precision, a small amount of light will eventually leak out of the optical cavity and be emitted tangentially from the internal surfaces of the micromirrors. Light emission from the side of the cavity has been frequently observed in many experiments with microcavity lasers [50,51].

We carried out lasing experiments to demonstrate the function of the microfluidic laser. A syringe needle was used to fill the microfluidic chamber with laser dye Rh6G dissolved in ethanol (~0.02 mol/L).

The microfluidic laser was then attached to an optical alignment stage and pumped by a pulsed, frequency-doubled Nd:YAG laser with a pulse duration of 5 ns and a repetition rate of 15 Hz. When the pumping power was increased above the lasing threshold, light emission could be clearly observed from the output end of the dye microlaser, as shown in Figure 23(a). We then placed a receiving screen approximately 8 mm from the output end of the structure to take a photograph of the far-field pattern of the emission, as shown in Figure 23(b). Two laser beams emitted tangentially from the internal surfaces of the two 45° mirrors were simultaneously observed on the screen, with one propagating upward and the other downward. The laser beams were well confined in the direction perpendicular to the plane of the optical cavity.

We measured the emission spectra of the microfluidic laser at different pumping energies. The detector head of the spectrometer (USB2000, Ocean Optics, Inc.) was placed near the output end of the microfluidic laser to collect the light from the beam that propagated downward. After measuring each spectrum, a power meter (Lasermate, Coherent, Inc.) was used to measure the average power of the pumping laser.

When a low pumping pulse fluence of 0.46 mJ/cm^2 was applied, only spontaneous emission with a broad spectrum was observed. Lasing commenced near a pumping fluence of 1.66 mJ/cm^2. Further increasing the pumping fluence greatly increased the output power of the microfluidic laser and narrowed its bandwidth. A typical emission spectrum of the microfluidic laser with a center wavelength of ~578 nm under a high pumping energy of 4.49 mJ/cm^2 was obtained with a bandwidth of approximately 5 nm. The output power of the microfluidic laser was evaluated at this pumping energy; the measured average power of one beam reached ~10 µW at a repetition rate of 15 Hz. Thus, a conservative estimate of the total pulse energy of both beams emitted from the microfluidic laser is approximately 1 µJ.

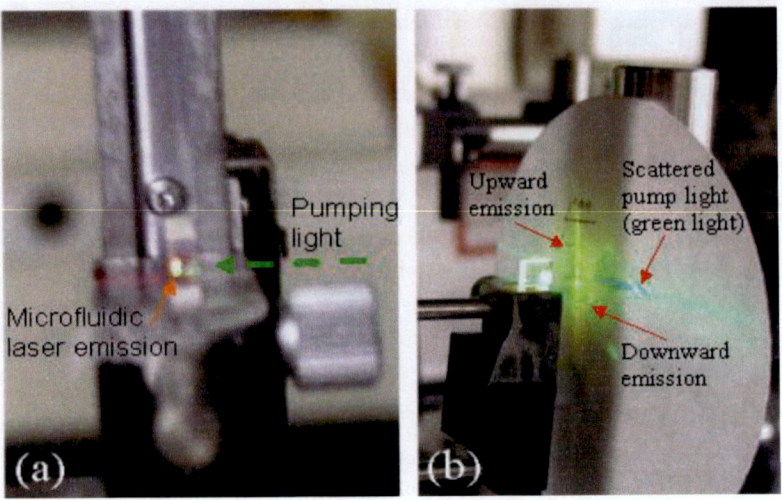

Figure 23. Digital camera images of (a) laser emission from glass sample and (b) far-field pattern of the laser beam on a receiving screen.

4.2. OPTOFLUIDIC INTEGRATION

In fact, the above-mentioned microfluidic dye laser is just one example of the general concept of optofluidic integration [54,55]. Toward this end, optical waveguides have been buried in Foturan glass by modifying its refractive index using femtosecond laser pulses, as described in Section 3.3 [38,39]. Additionally, optical waveguides and other microoptics such as microlenses and microfluidics can be easily integrated in a single glass chip by a single ultrafast laser system for manufacturing microchips for biochemical analysis and medical inspection. Such integrated microchips are often called optofluidics. Figure 26 shows a schematic illustration of a 3D integrated optofluidic system for photonic biosensing, in which one 6-mm-long optical waveguide is connected to a microfluidic chamber with dimensions of 1.0 mm × 1.0 mm × 1.0 mm, and two microlenses with a radius of curvature of 0.75 mm are separately arranged on the left side of the microchamber for fluorescence measurements and on the opposite side from the optical waveguide across the microchamber for absorption measurements with a distance of 300 μm. The inset shows an optical microscope image of the fabricated microchip. Experimental demonstration of photonic biosensing using the integrated microchip revealed that fluorescence analysis and absorption measurement of liquid samples can be performed with efficiencies enhanced by factors of 8 and 3, respectively [56].

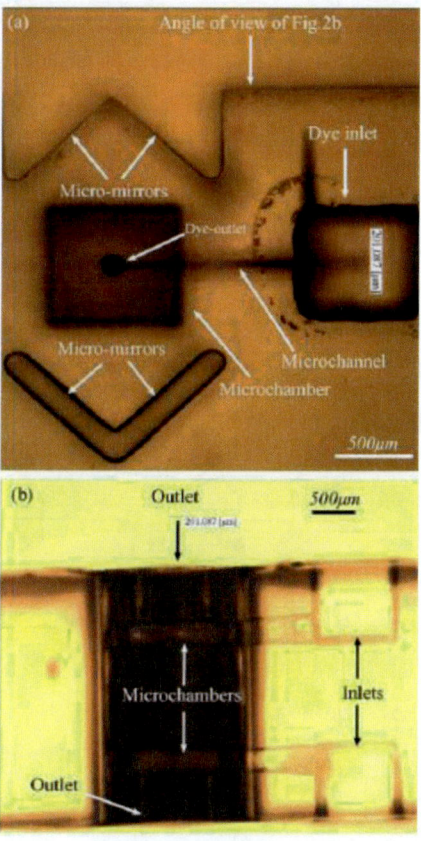

Figure 24. Optical micrographs of (a) top view of the dual-wavelength microfluidic laser and of (b) the side view of the two microfluidic chambers serially embedded in glass with a center-to-center distance of ~1000 mm.

In the examples below, the waveguides have to be written into the Foturan glass after fabricating micromirrors and microlenses, because the refractive index changes induced by femtosecond laser irradiation cannot withstand the high temperature applied to the Foturan sample during postannealing. This problem can easily be resolved by fabricating freestanding optical fibers rather than buried optical waveguides [57].

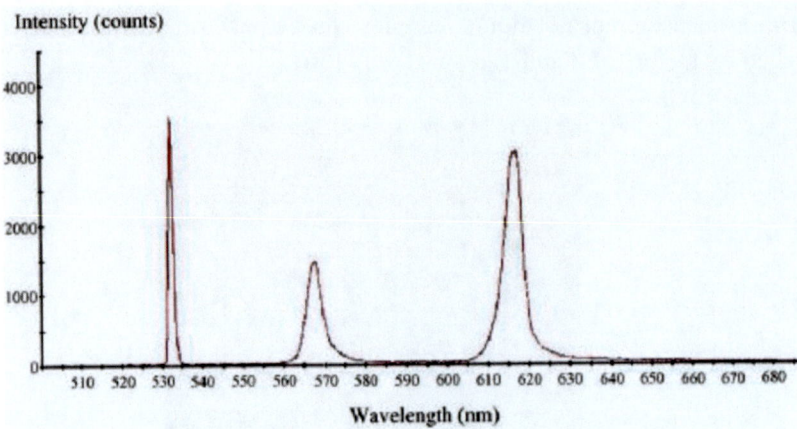

Figure 25. The spectrum of the dual-wavelength microfluidic laser. The peaks centered at 532, 568, and 618 nm correspond to scattered light from the pump laser, the Rh6G dye laser, and the rhodamine 640 dye laser, respectively.

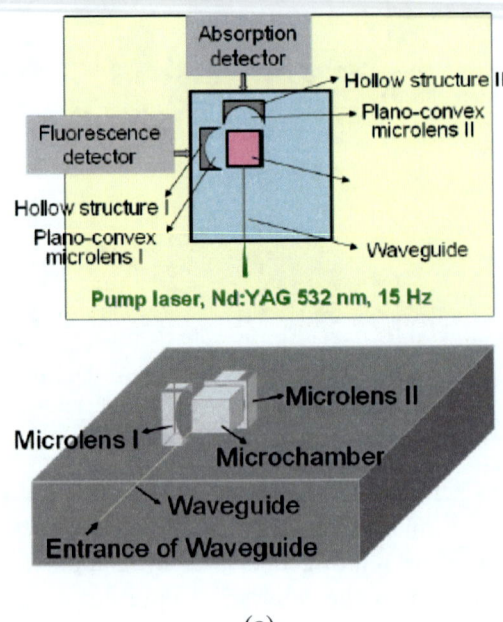

(a)

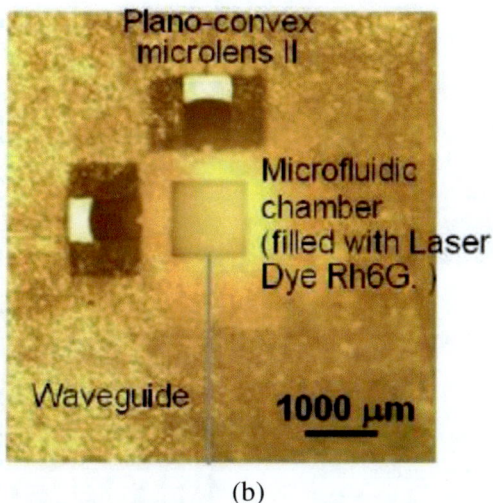

(b)

Figure 26. Schematic configuration of optofluidics in which microoptics, such as microoptical plano-convex lenses and an optical waveguide, are integrated with a microfluidic chamber in a single glass chip. An optical microscope image of the top view of the fabricated microchip is shown in the upper left corner.

A freestanding fiber was fabricated by scanning the area surrounding the fiber in a glass chip and then baking and etching the glass sample as described above. Figure 27(a) shows a structure composed of a freestanding fiber integrated with a 45° micromirror at the entrance of the fiber in the glass. The arrows in Figure 27(a) indicate the optical path of the coupling scheme. The 45° micromirror allows us to couple the light into the fiber from the side of the sample.

Figure 27(b) shows the optical micrograph of the micromirror and entrance of the fiber. The inset of Figure 27(b) (upper right corner) shows the cross-sectional shape of the fabricated fiber, which has approximate dimensions of 100 μm (width) × 80 μm (height). Light was coupled into the fiber by focusing a He-Ne laser beam on the micromirror using an objective lens with an NA of 0.46, as shown in Figure 27(c). The guided light was clearly observed at exit of the fiber. The total length of the fiber in Figure 27(c) is 8 mm, which is sufficiently long for many microchip applications. Fabricating longer fibers is not technically challenging, but it requires longer fabrication times. The measured loss for the freestanding fibers was approximately 1.3 dB/cm.

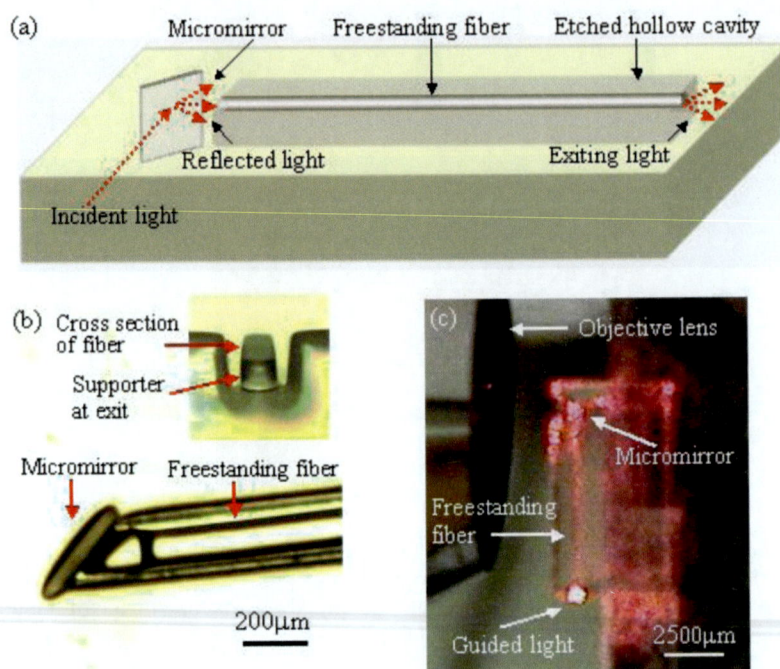

Figure 27. (a) 3D schematic drawing of a freestanding optical fiber integrated with a micromirror fabricated on a glass chip. Red arrows indicate the optical path of the coupling scheme. (b) Optical micrograph of the top view of the freestanding fiber and the micromirror. The inset (upper right corner) shows the cross-section of the fabricated fiber. (c) Digital-camera image of the side coupling of a HeNe laser beam into the freestanding fiber through the micromirror.

The freestanding fibers were then incorporated into a microfluidic circuit for on-chip biophotonic applications. Figure 28(a) illustrates a 3D schematic view of the integrated structure, which is a biosensor composed of two series of freestanding fibers intercepted by a microwell fabricated on a glass chip. Figure 28(b) shows an optical micrograph of part of the fabricated microstructure, showing the fibers and the microwell on the glass surface. To demonstrate that the light exiting from the first fiber can be effectively coupled into the second fiber, we focused the HeNe laser beam onto the entrance facet of the first fiber using a ×20 objective lens. As shown in Figure 28(c), both scattering light at the microwell and the exiting light at the end of the second fiber can clearly be observed. The coupling loss between the two fibers intercepted by the microwell was approximately 1 dB. We ascribe such a low coupling loss between the two fibers to two main factors: (1) the relatively large diameter of the fiber permits light beams with large mode areas to propagate in the fiber, thereby reducing the divergence angle of the exiting light, and (2) the inner walls of the microchannel between the two fibers are smooth and fabricated nearly perpendicular to the fibers, preventing the wavefront for the beam exiting the first fiber and entering the second fiber from tilting.

A freestanding fiber fabricated on a Foturan glass chip has many potential applications besides functioning as a waveguiding element. For example, the fiber could be fabricated inside a microfluidic channel and immersed in the sample solution. By measuring the optical loss of the beam propagating in the fiber, high-sensitivity photoabsorption measurements could be conducted. Moreover, because of the large refractive index difference between the freestanding fiber and the surrounding air, curved fibers can be fabricated with tight bends without significant optical losses.

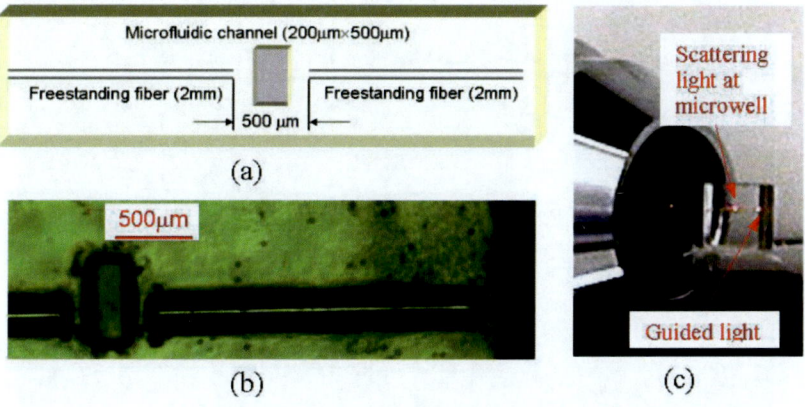

Figure 28. (a) Schematic 3D diagram of two freestanding optical fibers intercepted by a microwell fabricated on a glass chip. (b) Optical micrograph of the structure. (c) Image of the guiding He–Ne light through the entire structure. Scattering light at microwell and the guided light at the exit facet of the second fiber are indicated by arrows.

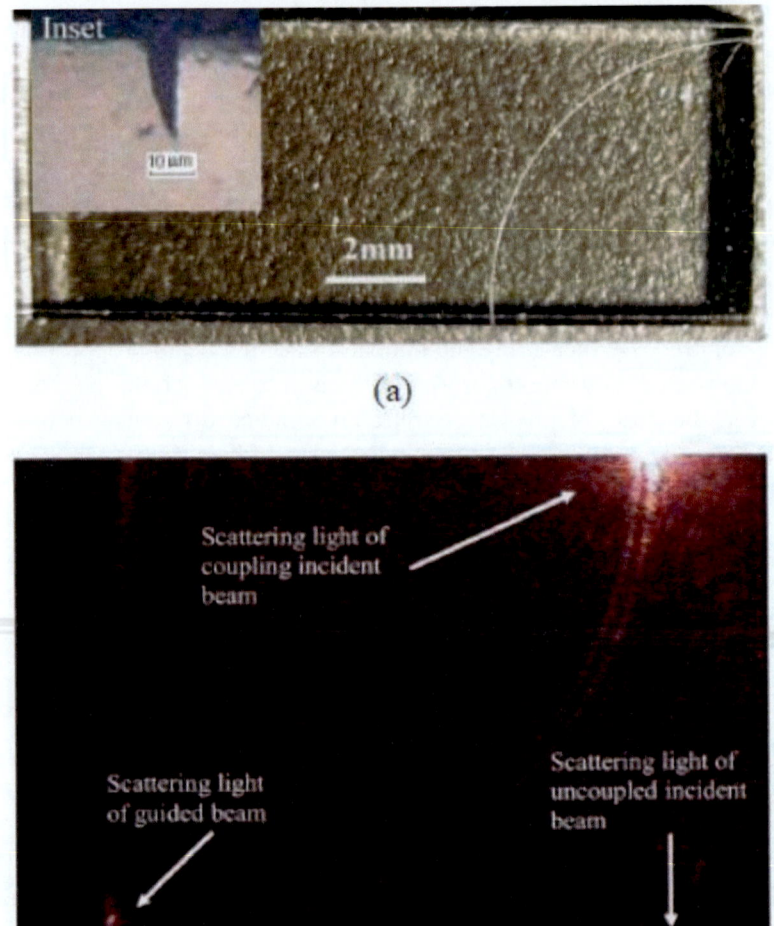

Figure 29. (a) Digital camera captured image of a 90° arc-shaped microchannel with a radius of curvature of 5 mm fabricated on a glass plate. Inset: cross-sectional view of the waveguide. (b) CCD camera image of the microfluidic optical waveguide carrying a He–Ne laser beam..

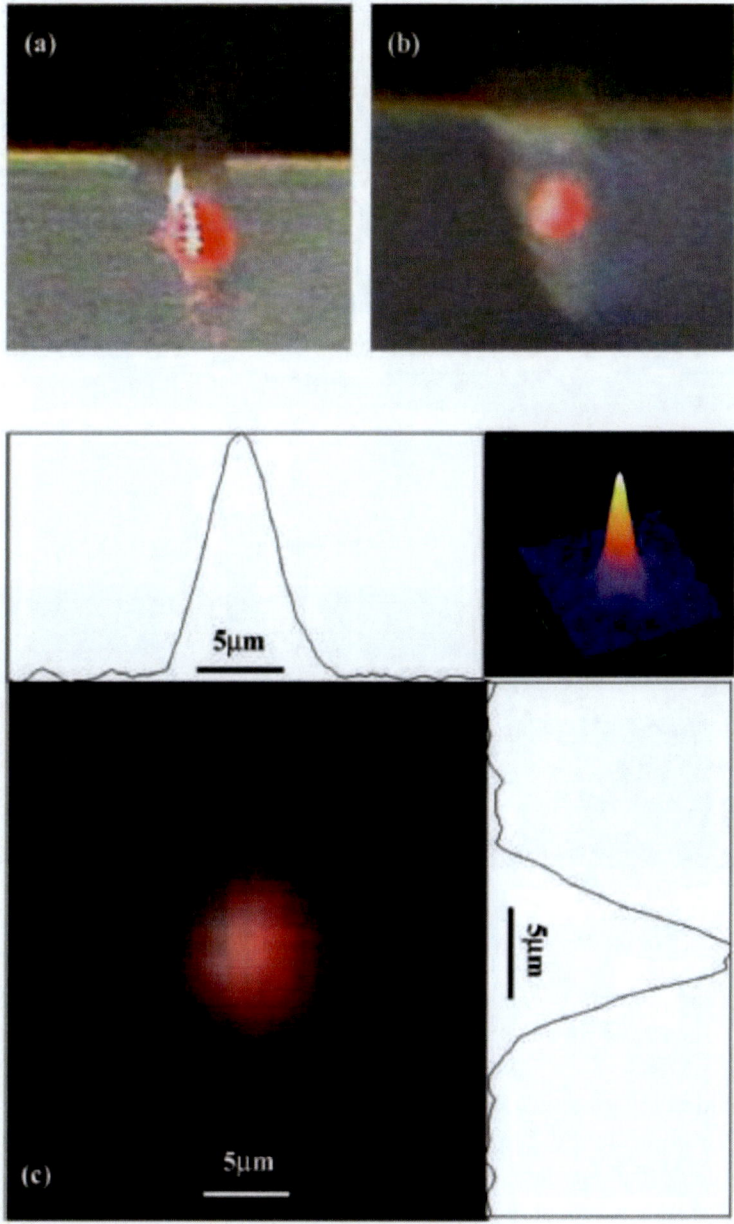

Figure 30. Near-field patterns of (a) multimode and (b) single-mode beams. (c) Beam profile of the single-mode beam.

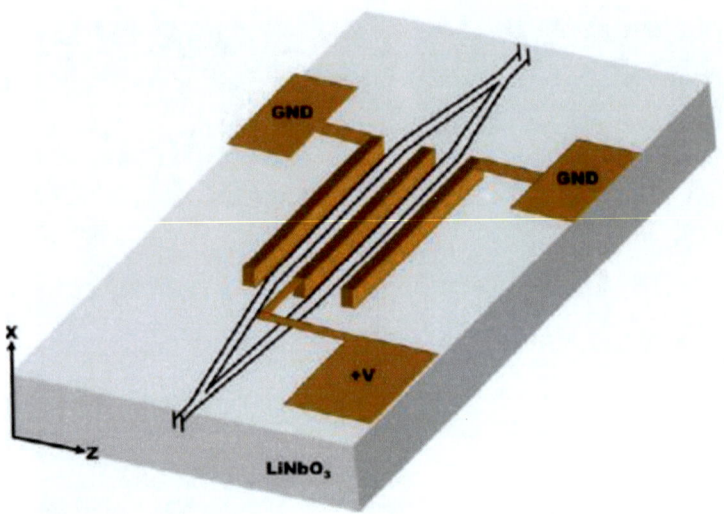

Figure 31. Schematic layout of the EO modulator.

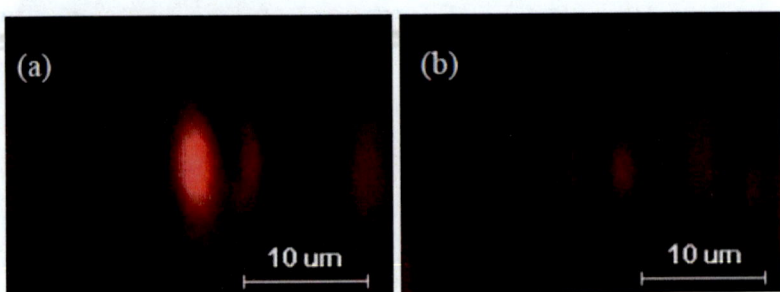

Figure 32. Near-field intensity distribution measured at the exit of EO modulator at dc voltages of (a) 0 V and (b) 19 V.

Recently, it has been pointed out that the curved freestanding fibers may find applications in astrophotonics (e.g., 3D mode converters in giant telescopes) [58].

Besides integrating individual fluidic and optical components in a single microchip, optofluidic chips can also be produced by employing microfluids as tunable optical media. One example of this is a microfluidic waveguide uses a liquid as the waveguide cores [59-62]. **Microfluidic waveguides can easily be fabricated by filling a microfluidic channel formed on a glass surface by femtosecond laser ablation with a liquid that has an adjustable refractive index** [59]. Figure 29(a) shows a digital camera image of a 90° arc-shaped microchannel with a radius of curvature of 5 mm fabricated on a glass plate. A cross-sectional view of the waveguide is shown in the inset; it shows a V-shaped channel with a width of ~7 μm at the opening and a depth of ~10 μm. Figure 29(b) shows a top view of the microfluidic optical waveguide carrying a He–Ne laser beam. Figure 30 shows end views of microfluidic waveguides carrying a HeNe laser beam. It can be seen that using the same microfluidic channel, the waveguide can be switched between multimode (Figure 30(a)) and single-mode operation (Figure 30(b)). This was achieved by using a mixture of two liquids (paraffin, n=1.474, and α-bromnaphtalene, n=1.658) with different refractive indices so that the refractive index can be tuned by varying the mixing ratio of the two liquids. In Figure 30(a), the refractive index of the liquid core was set to be 1.658, which can act as a multimode waveguide; while the refractive index was reduced to 1.527, which led to the formation of a single-mode waveguide as shown in Figure 30(b). Figure 30(c) shows a single-mode beam profile with a diameter of ~5 μm.

4.3. ELECTRO-OPTIC INTEGRATION

Although optofluidic integration by femtosecond laser direct writing is currently under intense investigation [63–65], electro-optic (EO) integration by the same approach has not been widely demonstrated to date. EO integration in transparent materials can be achieved by combining selective metallization and waveguide writing by focused femtosecond laser beam irradiation [45]. An excellent material for demonstrating EO integration is a lithium niobate ($LiNbO_3$) crystal, which is one of the most widely used nonlinear optical materials in integrated optics. Figure 31 shows a schematic diagram of a Mach–Zehnder interferometer (MZI) EO modulator is presented in. Commercially available MgO-doped x-cut $LiNbO_3$ crystals were used in the experiment. To produce thermally stable waveguides in the low repetition rate regime, we wrote two parallel lines with a close separation, which produced a guiding region between the two lines [66]. Unlike waveguides formed in the focal volume, a waveguide between the two tracks of the laser modified areas can preserve the nonlinearity of the bulk crystal [67]. Three embedded electrodes were integrated into the $LiNbO_3$ crystal, as illustrated in Figure 31. In addition, three metallic pads and connecting lines, which allow the modulator to be connected to an external electrical source, were fabricated together with the microelectrodes by the same technique.

The device was examined using a 633-nm He–Ne laser polarized in the extraordinary (Z) direction by applying a varying dc voltage to the electrodes, and we simultaneously captured images of the near-field mode at the output end of the MZI using a CCD camera. The results are shown in Figure 32. The measured extinction ratio was ~9.2 dB. A higher extinction ratio is expected if the two arms of the MZI can be fabricated more symmetrically by improving the translation precision of the XYZ stage. The voltage required to completely switch the modulator on and off was measured to be ~19 V, indicating an excellent EO overlap integral of ~0.95 [68].

The examples listed in this section demonstrate the potential of 3D femtosecond laser direct writing to integrate several fundamentally different functions in a single substrate. To our knowledge, there is currently no other continuous processing technique that offers the same capability.

Chapter 5

NANOAQUARIUM FOR DYNAMIC OBSERVATION OF MICROORGANISMS

5.1. CONCEPT OF NANOAQUARIUM

One important application of microfluidic structures embedded in Foturan glass fabricated by the present technique is the dynamic observation of microorganisms. A large variety of microorganisms live on the earth. Some of them move extremely rapidly, which is unusual in the macro-scale world in which we live, and exhibit unique 3D movement that goes against gravity. Most of them are single cells. It is very important to investigate their dynamic movement and physiological energy generation mechanisms to gain a better understanding of the potential ability and function of single cells that make up more complex organisms such as humans. The results will also be useful for developing biomotors. Consequently, observing microorganisms is currently important for cell biologists.

Optical microscopes equipped with high-speed cameras are commonly used by cell biologists to observe microorganisms [69-72]. In conventional observation systems, a glass slide with a coverslip or a Petri dish is generally used. However, the high-NA objective lens typically used for these observations limits the field of view to several hundred micrometers and it also restricts the depth of focus to several hundred micrometers, making it difficult to capture images of rapidly moving microorganisms. Consequently, it takes a very long time to obtain clear images of moving microorganisms. Reduced observation times are urgently needed by biologists not only in the interests of cost and time effectiveness, but also because of limited computer memory, which becomes problematic when acquiring movies using high-speed cameras.

To solve these problems, we propose using microchips with 3D microfluidic structures for observing microorganisms [32]. The microchip reduces the size of observation area; that is, it can three-dimensionally encapsulate microorganisms in a limited area. But it still provides sufficient space for them to move, making it much easier to capture images of their movement, as shown in Figure 33. Using a microchip in which microfluidics are three-dimensionally confined in glass has an additional advantage of enabling microorganisms to remain highly active for a long time, since such a structure prevents evaporation and leakage of water.

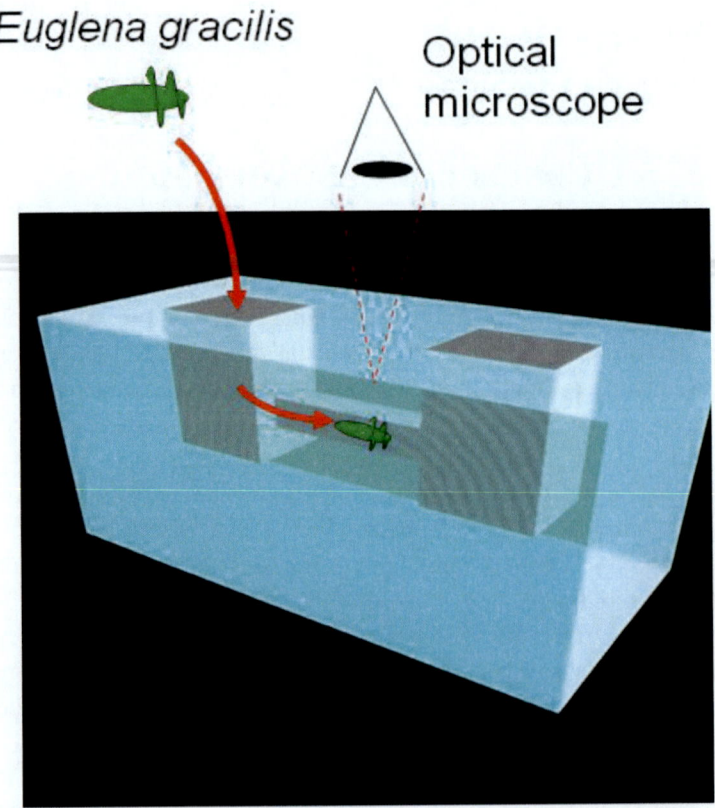

Figure 33. Concept of nanoaquarium for dynamic observation of microorganisms.

One advantage of our technique for fabricating 3D hollow microstructures is that a wide variety of structures can easily be fabricated by the same procedure, because of its ability to manufacture rapidly. The ability to rapidly manufacture various microchips with different structures and functions is needed by biologists to enable them to observe different kinds of microorganisms [73–76]. In addition, micromechanical components such as microvalves can be integrated in the microfluidics, as described in Section 3.2. Such functional microcomponents need to be integrated into microchips for some kinds of microorganisms (e.g., to stimulate a cell using a micromechanical component). Such functional microcomponents can be easily integrated by our technique. We refer to such microchips for observing microorganisms as nanoaquariums, because they are far smaller than conventional aquariums (although the microchannel widths in the microchips are of the order of several tens of microns). In addition, the volume of water used in such microchips is of the order of a nanoliter.

5.2. NANOAQUARIUM FOR OBSERVING THE MOTION OF EUGLENA GRACILIS

Euglena gracilis is a single-celled organism that lives in fresh water. It has a flagellum that emerges from the anterior end of the cell and it whips its flagellum rapidly to swim in water. Many biologists have used microscopes to investigate the continuous flagellum movement for both biomotor applications and to determine the origins of this functionality. However, only the thrusting movement of the flagellum has been investigated in previous research [77,78] and its detailed mechanism still remains unknown due to difficulties in capturing continuous high-speed images of the flagellum.

To enable clear and efficient observation of flagellum movement, we fabricated a microchannel in photosensitive glass, as depicted schematically in Figure 33. One *Euglena gracilis* is about 100 μm long and 40 μm wide and it generally propels itself forward by whipping its flagellum around its body. Therefore, we fabricated a microstructure with a 1-mm-long channel and with a cross-section of 150 μm × 150 μm embedded 150 μm below the glass surface. At both ends of the channel, two open reservoirs with dimensions of 500 μm × 500 μm were connected to allow the introduction of *Euglena gracilis* in water. The most important constraint in fabricating this microchip is that the distance between the glass surface and the upper wall of the microchannel needs to be between 130 μm and 170 μm, as determined by the working distance of the objective lens used for the observation. In this experiment, this distance was designed to be 150 μm. Furthermore, the etched glass surface must be smooth and the upper wall of the channel must be flat and parallel to the glass surface to obtain clear images. For observations, a *Euglena gracilis* is introduced into one of the reservoirs using an injection syringe filled with water. The microchannel is immediately filled with water and the *Euglena gracilis* swims into the microchannel by itself since there is no water flow in the microchannel. In the microchannel, the *Euglena gracilis* is confined in a limited area enabling dynamic observations of the flagellum movement to be performed easily using a microscope above the glass surface, as shown in Figure 33.

For microchip fabrication, the laser beam was translated in the glass sample line-by-line with a pitch of 5 μm and layer-by-layer with a pitch of 10 μm. After etching for 30 min in a 10% HF solution, additional heat treatment was performed to smooth the etched surface. This smoothing process is essential for obtaining clear images of *Euglena gracilis* in microscopic observations. Figure 34(a) shows optical micrographs of the top view of the microchip, and Figure 34(b) shows the side view of the microchannel when cutting the microchip along the dashed line indicated in Figure 34(a). As Figure 34(a) shows, a 1-mm-long microchannel with an almost constant width of 150 μm was fabricated. Figure 34(b) reveals that the microchannel has a rectangular cross-section and is embedded 150 μm below the glass surface, which satisfies the requirements for observations. In addition, the top internal wall of the microchannel is flat and smooth and is parallel to the glass surface. Such an internal wall was fabricated by multiple scanning of the laser beam with lateral shifts and additional annealing.

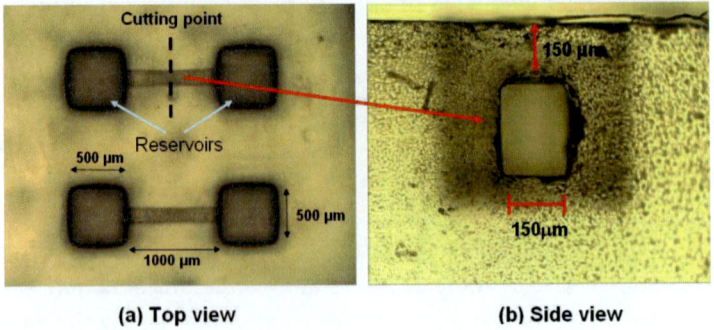

Figure 34. Optical microscope images of (a) the top view and (b) the side view of the microchip used for observing the motion of *Euglena gracilis*.

Figure 35(a) shows an optical microscope image of *Euglena gracilis* swimming in the embedded microchannel using the scheme shown in Figure

33. We also succeeded in recording movies, and Figure 35(b) shows enlarged sequential images of an advancing *Euglena gracilis* obtained from a movie. It shows that the *Euglena gracilis* coils its flagellum around its body and rotates very rapidly to swim in a straight line.

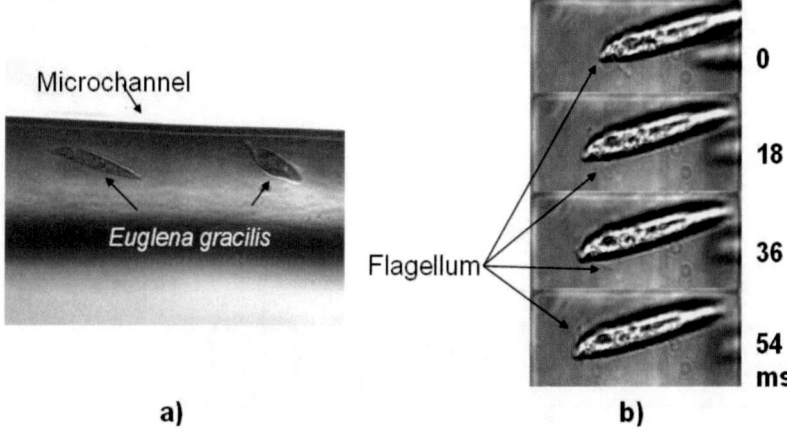

Figure 35. Microscope images of (a) encapsulated *Euglena gracilis* swimming in the microchannel and (b) sequential pictures of advancing *Euglena gracilis*.

Using this microchannel, we could stimulate the *Euglena gracilis* by irradiating light from any direction, and by this means we could easily control its motion. Figure 36(a) shows sequential pictures of a rotating *Euglena gracilis* when white light was irradiated from the bottom of the microchip, as shown in Figure 36(b). The *Euglena gracilis* turns its body to get away from the light since it is very sensitive to strong light. Interestingly, the *Euglena gracilis* thrust its flagellum forward to turn its body, unlike when it swims in a straight line (see Figure 36(b)). Furthermore, it has been impossible to observe *Euglena gracilis* from the front using conventional methods, although such observations are highly desirable for biologists to enable more detailed analysis of the flagellum movement. The microchip we developed enables such observations using the scheme shown in Figure 37(a). Figure 37(b) shows, for the first time, a front view of *Euglena gracilis* swimming upward in the reservoir, which is a part of a movie.

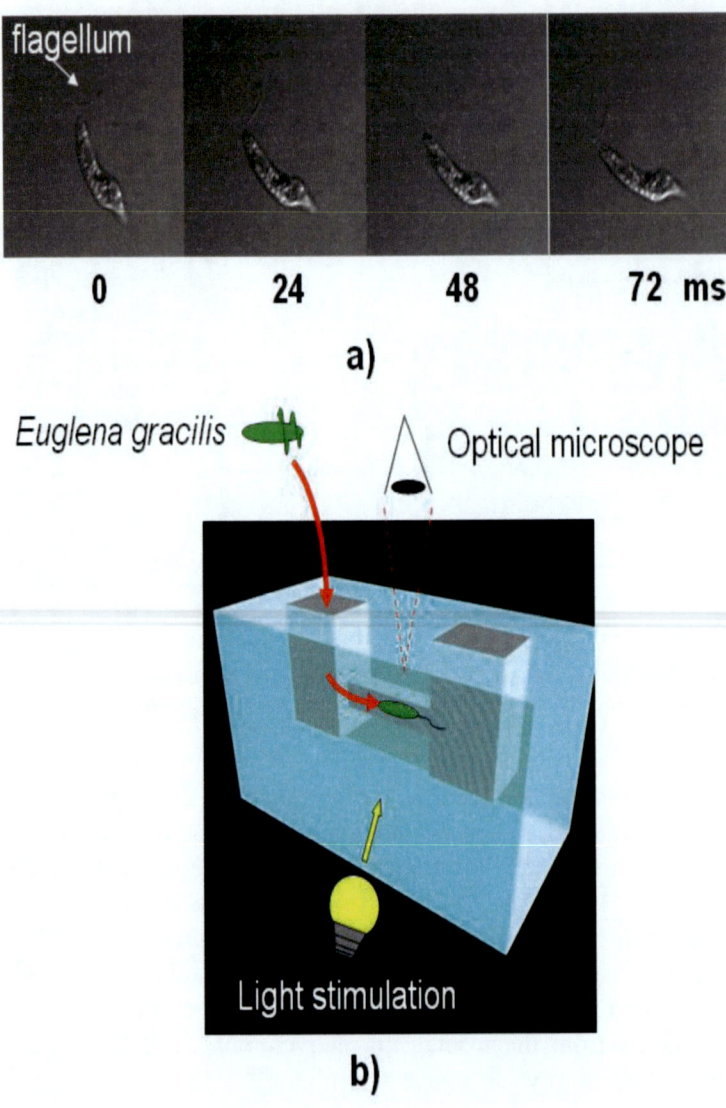

Figure 36. (a) Sequential pictures of rotating *Euglena gracilis* stimulated by light and (b) schematic illustration of the light stimulation of *Euglena gracilis* in the microchip.

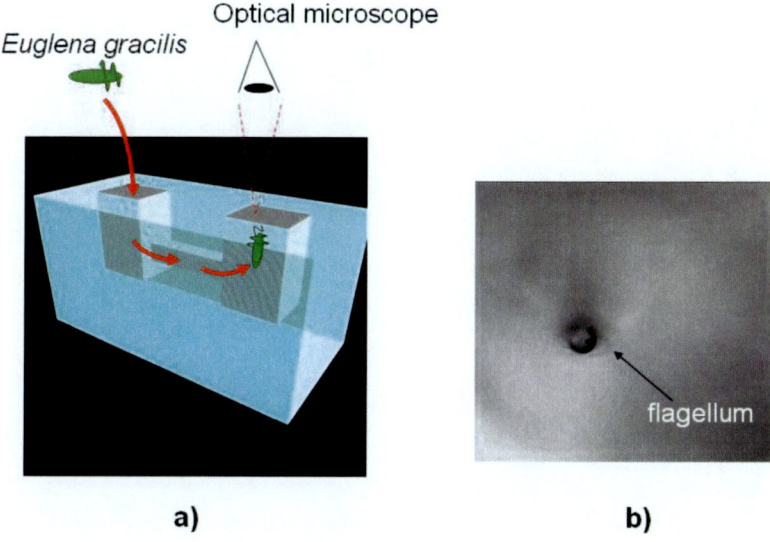

Figure 37. (a) Schematic illustration of the scheme for observing *Euglena gracilis* from the front and (b) microscopic image of the front view of *Euglena gracilis* swimming upward in the reservoir.

Using the microchip, the observation time can be reduced by a factor of more than 10 compared to the conventional method that uses a Petri dish. In addition, water in the embedded channel does not evaporate or leak, unlike when using a Petri dish, bonded glass, or polymer microchips.

Consequently, quantitative analysis of the flagellum movement could be easily carried out using the fabricated microchip. We have also succeeded in fabricating some other kinds of nanoaquariums with different structures and functionalities for various applications, including determining the information transmission process in *Pleurosira laevis*, observing the high-speed motion of Cryptomonas, and attaching Phormidium to seedling roots to promote the growth of Komatsuna.

Chapter 6

CONCLUSIONS AND OUTLOOK

As we have demonstrated above, we are currently able to obtain functions such as microfluidics, microoptics, photonics, micromechanics, and microelectronics in various transparent materials by 3D femtosecond laser direct writing. These functions can also be integrated into microchips to construct hybrid microdevices. A few integrated microfluidic biochips have been successfully used in biological research and they have important advantages over conventional techniques. All these facts clearly indicate that this technique has great potential to become an important tool for manufacturing LOC devices.

Although the examples given above make it appear straightforward to integrate functional components by 3D femtosecond laser direct writing, this is often not the case. The major difficulties that we currently face are as follows:

> Creation of embedded microfluidic channels and chambers inevitably requires chemical wet etching, while a limited contrast ratio in etching rates between modified and unmodified regions results in inhomogeneity in the microstructures (they are usually wider at openings and narrower in the middle). This problem becomes particularly severe when the channels are long. Thus, the lengths of most microfluidic structures produced by femtosecond laser direct writing followed by chemical etching are limited to a few millimeters or less, which is not sufficiently long for some LOC applications.
>
> The optical properties of microoptical components are still relatively poor compared to those of finely polished optical components fabricated by conventional techniques. For example, although over a small area (i.e., 20 μm × 20 μm), the average

roughness on an optical surface created by femtosecond laser direct writing can be as low as ~0.8 nm, the surface is still slightly wavy over a larger scale (e.g., a few hundred microns). As a result, a microlens fabricated by femtosecond laser direct writing followed by chemical etching and postannealing creates a significantly larger focal spot than the diffraction-limited one. This aspect certainly needs to be improved.

The compatibility of the fabrication procedures for different functional components requires further optimization, because it determines the ability to integrate certain elements. For example, in the fabrication of Foturan glass, postannealing after laser irradiation is required to develop a chemically etchable phase in the glass matrix. This will be unacceptable if it is desired to write an optical waveguide in glass by inducing refractive index changes in glass while simultaneously writing hollow structures. To overcome this problem, a waveguide can be written after forming all the hollow structures, but this solution means that fabrication is no longer be a single continuous process.

Because of the chemical etching procedure involved, the spatial resolution of this technique is of the order of micrometers. This urgently requires improvement. This is particularly important for microdevices integrated with microoptics. As is well known, for optical applications such as imaging or beam focusing, the positioning precision of lens should be on the wavelength scale or even better. It is very difficult to meet this requirement because of the uncertainty in removing glass material in the chemical etching process. Fortunately, optofluidic components are usually tunable so that this problem can be overcome by exploiting tunability.

Although the above-mentioned difficulties exist, we are optimistic that they can all be overcome by technical advances in the near future. At this stage, only microdevices integrated with a small number of elements have been successfully fabricated, such as the microfluidic laser, the nanoaquarium, and the microoptical modulator. However, we have started to fabricate more complex microdevices by femtosecond laser direct writing, which may eventually replace expensive and bulky equipment such as optical microscopes. The integration of microfluidics, microoptics, and microelectronics in a single glass chip may lead to active devices for applications in both biotechnology and information technology. Finally, we believe that close collaboration between physicists and biologists will lead to innovative devices that have never been previously fabricated being produced by 3D femtosecond laser direct writing.

REFERENCES

M. A. Burns, B. N. Johnson, S. N. Brahmasandra, K. Handique, J. R. Webster, M. Krishnan, T. S. Sammarco, P. M. Man, D. Jones, D. Heldsinger, C. H. Mastrangelo, and D. T. Burke, *Science*, 282, 484 (1998).
P. Yager, T. Edwards, E. Fu, K. Helton, K. Nelson, M. R. Tam and B. H. Weigl, *Nature*, 442, 412 (2006).
R. J. Jackman, T. M. Floyd, R. Ghodssi, M. A. Schmidt and K. F. Jensen, *J. Micromech. Microeng.* 11, 263 (2001).
Y. Xia, and G. M. Whitesides, *Annu. Rev. Mater. Sci.* 28, 153 (1998).
M. A. Unger, H. P. Chou, T. Thorsen, A. Scherer, and S. R. Quake, *Science*, 288, 113 (2000).
R. Gattass, and E. Mazur, *Nat. Photon.* 2, 219 (2008).
K. Sugioka, Y. Cheng, and K. Midorikawa, *Appl. Phys. A*, 81, 1 (2005).
H. Helvajian, P. D. Fuqua, W. W. Hansen, and S. Janson, *RIKEN Rev.* 32, 57 (2001).
Brabec, T. and Krausz, *Rev. Mod. Phys.* 72, 545 (2000).
M. Gertsvolf, H. Jean-Ruel, P. P. Rajeev, D. D. Klug, D. M. Rayner, and P. B. Corkum, *Phys. Rev. Lett.* 101, 243001 (2008).
Y. Cheng, K. Sugioka, M. Masuda, K. Toyoda, M. Kawachi, K. Shihoyama, and K. Midorikawa, RIKEN Rev. 50, 101 (2003).
See http://www.mikroglas.com/foturane.htm.
Stooky, "Photosensitively opacifiable glass," U.S. Patent 2684911 (1954).
M. Masuda, K. Sugioka, Y. Cheng, N. Aoki, M. Kawachi, K. Shihoyama, K. Toyoda, H. Helvajian, and K. Midorikawa, *Appl. Phys. A*, 76, 857, (2003).
Y. Kondo, J. Qiu, T. Mistsuyu, K. Hirao, and T. Yoko, Jpn. *J. Appl. Phys.* 38, L1146-1148 (1999).
T. Hongo, K. Sugioka, H. Niino, Y. Cheng, M. Masuda, I. Miyamoto, H. Takai, K. Midorikawa, *J. Appl. Phys.* 97, 063517 (2005).
Y. Cheng, K. Sugioka, K. Midorikawa, M. Masuda, K. Toyoda, M. Kawachi, and K. Shihoyama, *Opt. Lett.* 28, 1144 (2003).

References

Y. Cheng, H. L. Tsai, K. Sugioka, and K. Midorikawa, *Appl. Phys. A*, 85, 11 (2006).

J. Qiu, M. Shirai, T. Nakaya, J. Shi, X. Jiang, and C. Zhu, *Appl. Phys. Lett.* 81, 3040 (2002).

Y. Cheng, K. Sugioka, M. Masuda, K. Shihoyama, K. Toyoda, and K. Midorikawa, *Opt. Express*, 11, 1809 (2003).

C. Monat, P. Domachuk, and B. J. Eggleton, *Nat. Photon.* 1, 106 (2007).

Y. Cheng, K. Sugioka, and K. Midorikawa, *Opt. Lett.* 29, 2007 (2004).

K. Sugioka, M. Masuda, T. Hongo, Y. Cheng, K. Shihoyama, and K. Midorikawa, *Appl. Phys. A*, 78, 815 (2004).

M. Masuda, K. Sugioka, Y. Cheng, T. Hongo, K. Shihoyama, H. Takai, I. Miyamoto, and K. Midorikawa, *Appl. Phys. A*, 78, 1029 (2004).

M. Ams, G. Marshall, D. Spence, and M. Withford, .*Opt. Express*, 13, 5676 (2005).

K. Moh, Y. Tan, X.-C. Yuan, D. Low, and Z. Li, *Opt. Express*, 13, 7288 (2005).

S. Sowa, W. Watanabe, T. Tamaki, J. Nishii, and K. Itoh, *Opt. Express*, 14, 291 (2006).

S. Ho, P. R. Herman, Y. Cheng, K. Sugioka, and K. Midorikawa, "Direct ultrafast laser writing of buried waveguides in Foturan glass," in Conference on Lasers and Electro-Optics (CLEO), Vol. 96 of OSA Trends in Optics and Photonics Series, (Optical Society of America, Washington, D.C., 2004), paper CThD6.

K. Sugioka, Y. Cheng, K. Midorikawa, F. Takase, and H. Takai, *Opt. Lett.* 31, 208 (2006).

H. B. Sun, Y. Xu, S. Juodkazis, K. Sun, M. Watanabe, S. Matsuo, H. Misawa, and J. Nishii, *Opt. Lett.* 26, 325 (2001).

S. Matsuo, S. Kiyama, Y. Shichijo, T. Tomita, S. Hashimoto, Y. Hosokawa and H. Masuhara, *Appl. Phys. Lett.* 93, 051107 (2008).

Y. Hanada, K Sugioka, H. Kawano, I. S. Ishikawa, A. Miyawaki and K. Midorikawa, *Biomed. Microdevices*, 10, 403 (2008).

E. Verpoorte, *Lab. Chip*, 3, 42N (2003).

K.W. Ho, K. Lim, B.C. Shim, J.H. Hahn, Anal. Chem. 77, 5160 (2005).

Z. Wang, K. Sugioka, Y. Hanada, and K. Midorikawa, *Appl. Phys. A*, 89, 951 (2008).

K. M. Davis, K. Miura, N. Sugimoto, and K. Hirao, *Opt. Lett.* 21, 1729 (1996).

F. He, H. Sun, M. Huang, J. Xu, Y. Liao, Z. Zhou, Y. Cheng, Z. Xu, K. Sugioka and K. Midorikawa, Appl. Phys. A, online first, DOI: 10.1007/s00339-009-5338-4.

Z. Wang, K. Sugioka, Y. Hanada, and K. Midorikawa, *Appl. Phys. A*, 88, 699 (2007).

V.R. Bhardwaj, E. Simova, P. B. Corkum, D.M. Rayner, C. Hantovsky, R.S. Taylor, B. Schreder, M. Kluge, J. Zimmer, *J. Appl. Phys.* 97, 0 831 021 (2005).
Y. Hanada, K. Sugioka, and K. Midorikawa, *Appl. Phys. A*, 90, 603 (2008).
K. Sugioka, T. Hongo, and H. Takai, *Appl. Phys. Lett.* 86, 171901 (2005).
J. Xu, Y. Liao, H. Zeng, Z. Zhou, H. Sun, J. Song, X. Wang, Y. Cheng, Z. Xu, K. Sugioka, and K. Midorikawa, *Opt. Express*, 15, 12743 (2007).
J. Xu, Y. Liao, H. Zeng, Y. Cheng, Zhizhan Xu, Koji Sugioka and Katsumi Midorikawa, *Opt. Commun.* 281, 3505 (2008).
Y. Liao, J. Xu, H. Sun, J. Song, X. Wang, and Y. Cheng, *Appl. Surf. Sci.* 254, 7018 (2008).
Y. Liao, J. Xu, Y. Cheng, Z. Zhou, F. He, H. Sun, J. Song, X. Wang, Z. Xu, K. Sugioka, and K. Midorikawa, Opt. Lett. 33, 2281 (2008).
L. Gui, B. Xi, and T.C. Chong, *IEEE Photonics Technol. Lett.* 16, 1337 (2004).
G. A. Shafeev, Appl. Phys. A 67, 303 (1998).
T. J. Hirsch, R. F. Miracky, and C. Lin, *Appl. Phys. Lett.* 57, 1357 (1990).
P. Joglekar, H. Liu, E. Meyhöfer, G. Mourou, and A. J. Hunt, *Proc. Natl. Acad. Sci. USA,* 101, 5856 (2004).
W. Poon, F. Courvoisier, and R. K. Chang, *Opt. Lett.* 26, 632 (2001).
H. J. Moon, Y. T. Chough, and K. An, *Phys. Rev. Lett.* 85, 3161 (2000).
Y. Cheng, K. Sugioka, and K. Midorikawa, *Appl. Surf. Sci.* 248, 172 (2005).
Q. Kou, I. Yesilyurt, and Y. Chen, *Appl. Phys. Lett.* 88, 091101 (2005).
D. Psaltis, S. R. Quake, C. H. Yang, *Nature,* 442, 381 (2006).
Y. Cheng, K. Sugioka, and K. Midorikawa, *Proc. SPIE*, 5662, 209 (2004).
Z. Wang, K. Sugioka, and K. Midorikawa, *Appl. Phys. A*, 93, 225 (2008).
Y. Cheng, K. Sugioka, K. Midorikawa, *Opt. Express*, 13, 7225 (2005).
R. R. Thomson, A. K. Kar, and J. Allington-Smith, *.Opt. Express,* 17, 1963 (2009).
H. Sun, F. He, Z. Zhou, Y. Cheng, Z. Xu, K. Sugioka, and K. Midorikawa, *Opt. Lett.* 32, 1536 (2007).
D. B. Wolfe, R. S. Conroy, P. Garstecki, B. T. Mayers, M. A. Fischbach, K. E. Paul, M. Prentiss, and G. M. Whitesides, *Proc. Natl. Acad. Sci. U.S.A.* 101, 12434 (2004).
P. Dumais, C. L. Callender, J. P. Noad, and C. J. Ledderhof, *IEEE Photon. Technol. Lett.* 18, 746 (2006).
M. Brown, T. Vestad, J. Oakey, and D. W. M. Marret, *Appl. Phys. Lett.* 88, 134109 (2006).
R. Osellame, V. Maselli, R. M. Vazquez, R. Ramponi, and G. Cerullo, *Appl. Phys. Lett.* 90, 231118 (2007).
V. Maselli, J. R. Grenier, S. Ho, and P. R. Herman, *Opt. Express,* 17, 11719 (2009).

M. Kim, D. J. Hwang, H. Jeon, K. Hiromatsu, and C. P. Grigoropoulos, *Lab Chip*, 9, 311 (2009).

J. Burghoff, C. Grebing, S. Nolte, and A. Tünnermann, *Appl. Phys. Lett.* 89, 081108 (2006).

J. Thomas, M. Heinrich, J. Burghoff, S. Nolte, A. Ancona, A. Tünnermann, *Appl. Phys. Lett.* 91, 151108 (2007).

L. N. Binh, *J. Cryst. Growth*, 288, 180 (2006).

K. Okano, E. Hunter, and N. Fusetani, *J. Exp. Zool.* 276, 138 (1996).

K. Yoshimura, C. Shingyoji, and K. Takahashi, Cell Motil. *Cytoskeleton*, 36, 236 (1997).

S.L. Fleming and C. L. Rieder, Cell Motil. Cytoskeleton 56, 141 (2003).

D. J. Stephens, and V. J. Allan, *Science*, 300, 82 (2003).

Yamahata, C. Vandevyver, F. Lacharme, P. Izewska, H. Vogel, R. Freitag, and M.A.M. Gijs, *Lab Chip*, 5, 1083 (2005).

Y. Choi, M.A. McClain, M.C. LaPlaca, A.B. Frazier, and M.G. Allen, Biomed. *Microdevices*, 9, 7 (2007).

S. Haeberle and R. Zengerle, *Lab Chip*. 7, 1094 (2007).

Funfak, A. Brösing, M. Brand, and J. M. Köhler, *Lab Chip*. 7, 1132 (2007).

K. M. Nichols, and R. Rikmenspoel, *J. Cell Sci.* 23, 211 (1977).

K. M. Nichols, and R. Rikmenspoel, *J. Cell Sci.* 29, 233 (1978).

INDEX

A

absorption, 2, 5, 9, 47
acetone, 39, 40
acid, 8, 11
adhesion, 37
AFM, 27
air, 16, 21, 22, 23, 29, 53
aluminosilicate, 8
aluminum, 44
amorphous, 8
annealing, 25, 26, 27, 30, 33, 66
application, 2, 37, 39, 61
applications, 2, 4, 16, 20, 25, 30, 35, 51, 52, 56, 64, 69, 72, 73
appropriate technology, 3
aqueous solution, 11
aspect ratio, 13, 15
atoms, 5, 8
automation, 2

B

baking, 11, 50
bandwidth, 46
beams, 16, 17, 18, 20, 31, 45, 46, 52, 55
bending, 36
binding, 6
biological behavior, 2
biosensors, 27
biotechnology, 73
bonding, 3, 12
broad spectrum, 46
bulk crystal, 58

C

cell, 17, 21, 61, 63, 64
cerium, 8
challenges, 2, 4
channels, 3, 11, 13, 16, 19, 71
charge coupled device, 7
chemical etching, 9, 12, 22, 24, 27, 72, 73
chemical properties, 6
clusters, 8
collaboration, 73
compaction, 33
compatibility, 72
complexity, 3
components, 1, 3, 4, 9, 11, 24, 30, 37, 56, 63, 71, 72, 73
concentration, 11

configuration, 13, 50
control, 67
convex, 29, 31, 35, 36, 50
copper, 37, 38, 39, 40
cost-effective, 42
coupling, 33, 34, 50, 52
cross-sectional, 19, 51, 54, 57
crystalline, 8
crystallites, 20, 25
crystals, 58

D

detection, 24, 43
dielectric materials, 37
dielectrics, 42
diffraction, 13, 31, 32, 72
distilled water, 24
distribution, 16, 18, 56
divergence, 25, 26, 52
doped, 8, 58
drawing, 51
duration, 5, 45
dynamics, 2

E

earth, 61
electric field, 5
electric power, 37
electrodes, 40, 58
electromagnetic, 5
electromagnetic wave, 5
electron, 8
electrons, 6, 8
emission, 45, 46, 47
encapsulated, 20, 67
energy, 5, 16, 18, 24, 30, 46, 61
equipment, 73
etching, 8, 9, 11, 21, 22, 24, 27, 50, 65, 71, 72, 73
ethanol, 45

evaporation, 62
excitation, 9
exposure, 8, 12, 20, 22
extinction, 58

F

fabricate, 3, 4, 8, 20, 24, 32, 41, 73
fabrication, ix, 2, 3, 6, 7, 9, 11, 20, 29, 38, 40, 42, 45, 51, 65, 72
fiber, 50, 51, 52, 53
fibers, 49, 51, 52, 53, 56
film, 37, 39
films, 38, 40
flagellum, 64, 66, 67, 69
flow, 21, 22, 24, 65
fluorescence, 17, 18, 43, 47
focusing, 6, 15, 16, 17, 29, 32, 51, 73
formula, 29
fresh water, 64

G

gas, 24
generation, 61
glasses, 14
gracilis, 64, 65, 66, 67, 68, 69
gravity, 61
growth, 2, 69

H

healthcare, 2
heat, 6, 8, 24, 65
height, 13, 51
helium, 24
high temperature, 48
high-speed, 61, 64, 69
humans, 61
Hunter, 78
hybrid, 2, 3, 43, 71
hydrofluoric acid, 8

I

ideal, 1, 9
illumination, 16
image, 35, 36, 39, 47, 50, 52, 54, 57, 66, 69
images, 11, 27, 28, 29, 31, 35, 37, 38, 40, 47, 58, 62, 64, 65, 66, 67
imaging, 27, 73
indices, 16, 30, 57
industry, 2
information technology, 73
inhomogeneity, 71
injection, 65
inspection, 47
insulators, 40, 41
integrated circuits, ix, 1
integrated optics, 58
integration, 1, 3, 4, 24, 35, 36, 39, 47, 57, 73
interaction, 1, 5, 9
interface, 29
interval, 24, 40
ions, 8
irradiation, 9, 16, 18, 19, 20, 21, 24, 27, 30, 48, 57, 72
isotropic, 16, 19

L

large-scale, 12
laser ablation, 37, 57
lasers, 5, 41, 45
lasing threshold, 45
leakage, 62
lens, 7, 11, 13, 27, 29, 30, 32, 35, 51, 52, 62, 65, 73
lenses, 9, 17, 28, 32, 50
light beam, 25, 36, 52
line, 65, 66, 67
linear, 6, 9, 33, 37
linear function, 37

liquids, 17, 57
lithium, 8, 20, 24, 39, 57
lithography, 1, 3
losses, 53

M

mainstream, 1
manufacturing, 2, 12, 47, 71
matrix, 8, 28, 72
measurement, 47
media, 56
medicine, 2
memory, 62
meter, 46
microcavity, 43, 45
microchip, 2, 35, 37, 47, 50, 51, 56, 62, 65, 66, 67, 68, 69
microelectrodes, 40, 41, 58
microelectronics, 1, 3, 71, 73
microfabrication, 1, 2, 3, 5, 8
microfluidic channels, 3, 11, 13, 16, 19, 71
microfluidic devices, 36
micrometer, 6
microorganisms, 2, 4, 61, 63
microscope, 29, 31, 35, 36, 37, 38, 39, 47, 50, 65, 66
microstructure, 15, 52, 64
microstructures, 1, 3, 7, 8, 16, 19, 28, 63, 71
microvoids, 16
miniaturization, 1
mixing, 16, 57
motion, 21, 66, 67, 69
movement, 61, 62, 64, 67, 69

N

nanoclusters, 8
nanodots, 26
nanometer, 6, 42

nanoparticles, 9, 30, 33
nanostructures, 42
national security, 3
neon, 24
network, 21, 25
nitrate, 38, 40
nitrogen, 24
nitrogen gas, 24
nuclei, 8
numerical aperture, 7

O

objectives, 6
observations, 62, 65, 67
one dimension, 32
online, 77
optical, 1, 9, 14, 16, 17, 18, 24, 26, 27, 29, 31, 32, 33, 34, 35, 36, 37, 40, 43, 44, 45, 47, 49, 50, 51, 52, 53, 54, 56, 58, 65, 66, 72, 73
optical fiber, 49, 51, 53
optical micrographs, 65
optical properties, 9, 24, 72
optics, 58
optimization, 72
order, 5, 35, 64, 73
organism, 64
OSA, 76
overlap, 16, 17, 58

P

packaging, 3
parallel, 13, 16, 24, 32, 58, 65
performance, 29
Petri dish, 62
photoabsorption, 43, 53
photochemical, 30
photographs, 22
photolithography, 3
photon, 8, 20

photonic, 20, 30, 47
photonics, 2, 71
photons, 6
physical properties, 35
physicists, 73
physiological, 61
pitch, 31, 32, 65
planar, 1
polymer, 69
polymerization, 20
poor, 9, 72
power, 37, 38, 40, 45, 46
production, 2
propagation, 9, 13, 33, 34, 36
properties, 25
property, 5
pulse, 5, 6, 24, 30, 32, 33, 45, 46
pulses, 5, 40, 47
pumping, 45, 46

R

radius, 29, 47, 54, 57
range, 2, 7, 20, 34
reactant, 12
reactions, 32
reagent, 2, 21
reagents, 21
reason, 5
recommendations, iv
reflection, 24, 44
refractive index, 7, 9, 16, 29, 30, 32, 35, 47, 48, 53, 57, 72
refractive indices, 16, 30, 57
region, 9, 16, 18, 30, 33, 58
reservoir, 67, 69
reservoirs, 64
resolution, 7, 9, 13, 19, 21, 30, 42, 73
robustness, 24
roughness, 25, 26, 37, 72
routing, 20

S

sample, 2, 7, 9, 11, 14, 16, 17, 20, 22, 24, 26, 32, 47, 48, 50, 52, 65
scattered light, 49
scattering, 25, 52
security, 3
SEM, 28
semiconductor, 3
sensitivity, 52
separation, 58
series, 52
shape, 13, 16, 29, 51
silica, 37
silicon, 1, 21
silver, 8, 9, 30, 33, 38, 40
smoothing, 65
smoothness, 26
soft lithography, 3
space, 7, 16, 62
spatial, 7, 21, 30, 42, 73
spectroscopy, 43
spectrum, 46, 49
speed, 16, 24, 32, 37, 38, 40, 61, 64, 69
stability, 24
standardization, 2
storage, 16, 20
structuring, 1
substrates, 3, 21, 38, 40
supply, 12
suppression, 6
surface roughness, 25, 26, 37
switching, 20
systems, 1, 3, 6, 37, 43, 61

T

technology, 1, 2, 73
temperature, 25, 37, 39, 48
thermal treatment, 35
thin film, 38, 40
thin films, 38, 40
three-dimensional, 16, 62
threshold, 2, 6, 21, 41, 45
time, 18, 32, 62, 67, 69
total internal reflection, 44
tracks, 58
trade, 7
trans, 16
translation, 17, 18, 58
transmission, 22, 33, 36, 37, 69
transparent, 1, 3, 4, 5, 7, 30, 57, 71

U

uncertainty, 73
uniform, 11
UV, 8, 12
UV exposure, 9, 12

V

values, 34
velocity, 20
visible, 29, 33

W

waste, 2
water, 24, 62, 64, 69
waveguide, 31, 33, 35, 36, 47, 50, 54, 56, 57, 72
wavelengths, 6
writing, 1, 2, 3, 4, 5, 6, 7, 8, 11, 14, 20, 28, 30, 31, 32, 35, 37, 38, 40, 43, 57, 58, 71, 72, 73, 76
writing process, 4

Y

yttrium, 44